Interventional Radiology for Medical Students

Hong Kuan Kok • Elizabeth Ryan
Hamed Asadi • Michael Lee
Editors

Interventional Radiology for Medical Students

Springer

Editors
Hong Kuan Kok
Department of Radiology
Beaumont Hospital and Royal College of Surgeons in Ireland
Dublin
Ireland

Hamed Asadi
Interventional Neuroradiology Service
Austin Health
Melbourne
Victoria
Australia

School of Medicine, Faculty of Health
Deakin University
Victoria
Australia

Elizabeth Ryan
Department of Radiology
Beaumont Hospital and Royal College of Surgeons in Ireland
Dublin
Ireland

Michael Lee
Department of Radiology
Beaumont Hospital and Royal College of Surgeons in Ireland
Dublin
Ireland

ISBN 978-3-319-53852-5 ISBN 978-3-319-53853-2 (eBook)
DOI 10.1007/978-3-319-53853-2

Library of Congress Control Number: 2017953047

Printed on acid-free paper

This Springer imprint is published by Springer Nature
The registered company is Springer International Publishing AG
The registered company address is: Gewerbestrasse 11, 6330 Cham, Switzerland

To my parents, Sonny and Karen; my wife, Limy; and my family, Adrian and Tiffany

– Hong Kuan Kok

To my family and colleagues for their much valued support and to all students of the wonderful field of Interventional Radiology

– Elizabeth Ryan

To my beautiful wife Anousha and our lovely Tara and Daniel

– Hamed Asadi

To Aoife, Ronan, Daire and Sarah

– Michael Lee

Foreword

IR has grown over the last forty years from a small cadre of enthusiasts who were on the outside of mainstream medicine to the current situation where IR is now an essential part of modern healthcare delivery. For any specialty, teaching the next generation of doctors is vitally important. It has been shown that medical students are much more likely to choose a career in a specialty if they have been taught or mentored by doctors within that specialty. As interventional radiology comes of age, dedicated IR teaching is a must for all medical schools so that qualified doctors are familiar with the scope of IR and can refer appropriately. This is even more important in the current era because of the rapid growth in the breadth and depth of IR procedures, which are used to treat a diverse group of diseases and conditions.

This book covers the main topics of interventional radiology in a case-based format for optimal learning and retention. Biopsy and drainage, angioplasty and stenting, embolisation, musculoskeletal IR and neuro intervention, including stroke thrombectomy, are all covered. The book has been edited and written by IR experts who have delivered the IR teaching programme at Beaumont Hospital over a number of years. It is our hope that this book will familiarize medical students, general practitioners and other interested parties with the dynamic specialty of IR and what IR can contribute to patient care.

We hope that you enjoy the book and through reading this book you will gain an understanding of modern IR practice and where it fits in hospital practice.

Dublin Ireland　　　　Michael Lee

Preface

Interventional radiology or "IR" has been practiced since 1954 when a Swedish radiologist called Sven Seldinger devised a system to puncture the femoral artery and gain access with a catheter to perform diagnostic angiography. This simple invention provided safe access to the arterial system and diagnostic radiology morphed into interventional radiology. IR has grown and matured since its inception, and in the last twenty years has become a vitally important part of patient care. In fact, for many diseases, one cannot receive appropriate care without using IR services.

As IR moves to becoming a specialty in its own right, it is important that IR take up its teaching duties and teaches the next generation of doctors. We decided to write this book because of the enthusiastic reception of IR teaching by medical students attached to RCSI (Royal College of Surgeons in Ireland) medical schools in Dublin, Bahrain and Malaysia. We have been teaching IR to our medical students in a dedicated curriculum for the past four years and this book is based on that experience. The book is in a case-based format, which we believe enhances the learning experience for medical students. All of the important topics in modern IR are covered.

As IR grows and attains specialist status in its own right we hope that IR teaching in medical schools will become the norm rather than the exception.

Dublin Ireland — Michael Lee

Contents

Contributors

Hamed Asadi, MD, PhD, FRANZCR, CCINR, EBIR Interventional Neuroradiology Service, Austin Health, Melbourne, Victoria, Australia

School of Medicine, Faculty of Health, Deakin University, Victoria, Australia

Mark F. Given, AFRCSI, FFR RCSI, EBIR Department of Radiology, Beaumont Hospital, Dublin, Ireland

Gareth Kiernan, MRCPI, FFR RCSI Department of Radiology, Beaumont Hospital, Dublin, Ireland

Hong Kuan Kok, MRCPI FFR RCSI FRCR EBIR Department of Radiology, Beaumont Hospital and Royal College of Surgeons in Ireland, Dublin, Ireland

Michael Lee, FRCPI FFR RCSI FRCR EBIR, FSIR Department of Radiology, Beaumont Hospital and Royal College of Surgeons in Ireland, Dublin, Ireland

Timothy Murray, MRCSI, FFR RCSI Department of Radiology, Beaumont Hospital, Dublin, Ireland

Damien O'Neill, MRCSI Department of Radiology, Beaumont Hospital, Dublin, Ireland

Elizabeth Ryan, MRCSI, FFR RCSI Department of Radiology, Beaumont Hospital and Royal College of Surgeons in Ireland, Dublin, Ireland

Mark Sheehan, MRCSI Department of Radiology, Beaumont Hospital and Royal College of Surgeons in Ireland, Dublin, Ireland

Introduction to Interventional Radiology

1

Mark Sheehan and Michael Lee

1.1 Introduction

- The field of medicine is constantly changing, evolving and outcomes for patients are improving with the increasing use of minimally invasive surgical techniques. Interventional Radiology (IR) or image guided minimally invasive surgery has demonstrated enormous innovation over the last 20 years and has developed multiple new minimally invasive alternatives to traditional surgical procedures.
- IR is now a must in all reasonably sized hospitals to ensure optimal patient care.
- The competent medical student needs to know:
  - The basic principles of IR.
  - The role of IR within clinical practice.
  - Image guidance techniques used in IR.
  - Consent and patient preparation for IR procedures.
  - Importance of radiation protection.

1.2 History of Interventional Radiology

- Since the Seldinger technique was first developed in 1953 by a Swedish radiologist of the same name, IR has made significant advancement. Some of the common procedural terms used in IR are listed below:
  - Angioplasty (opening an artery, vein or other tubular structure with a balloon),

M. Sheehan • M. Lee (✉)
Department of Radiology, Beaumont Hospital and Royal College of Surgeons in Ireland, Dublin, Ireland
e-mail: marksheehan@rcsi.ie

H.K. Kok et al. (eds.), *Interventional Radiology for Medical Students*,
DOI 10.1007/978-3-319-53853-2_1

- Stent placement (using a stent in an artery, vein or tubular structure to support angioplasty)
- Biopsy and Drainage - using image guidance to obtain a tissue or fluid sample to aid diagnosis or drain an abscess, obstructed biliary system (biliary drainage) or obstructed renal (nephrostomy) system
- Embolisation (blocking an artery that is bleeding, delivering payload to an artery supplying a tumor)
- Tumor ablation or Interventional Oncology (ablating or destroying tumours by using thermal energy).

- Charles Theodore Dotter, also known as the "Father of interventional radiology" performed the first angioplasty in 1964. Dr. Dotter later went on to receive a Nobel prize nomination in 1978 for the development of this procedure.
- In 1966 the first embolisation techniques were pioneered to treat tumours and spinal cord vascular malformations.
- In the 1970s embolisation of the arteries supplying the gastrointestinal (GI) tract was used to treat massive GI bleeds.
- In the 1980s, Transjugular Intrahepatic Portosystemic shunt (TIPS) was first used to treat life threatening variceal bleeding in patients with portal hypertension.
- In the early 90s, Endovascular aneurysm repair (EVAR) was first used to treat abdominal aortic aneurysms (AAA) and is now the preferred treatment for elective AAA repair.
- In the late 90s, the use of radiofrequency ablation for the treatment of varicose veins first began and its use is now widespread.
- The training of Interventional Radiologists has also evolved greatly over this time. Typically an IR trainee undertakes 3–4 years of basic Radiology training followed by at least two higher training (also known as Fellowship) years in IR.
- Training follows a national or supranational curriculum such as the CIRSE (Cardiovascular and Interventional Radiology Society of Europe) curriculum where trainees are expected to gain competency in the imaging, technical and clinical aspects of IR and patient management.
- Assessment of competency of IR training is now available in most jurisdictions through the European Board of Interventional Radiology (EBIR) in Europe, Australia and New Zealand, the Certificate of Added Qualification in Vascular & Interventional Radiology (CAQ in VIR) exam in the USA and examinations or continuous appraisal in other countries.

1.3 Patient Preparation and Safety Checklist

- Patient preparation for IR procedures is similar to patient preparation for surgical procedures.
- Informed consent must be obtained form all patients, preferably form the doctor performing the procedure or a delegate with suitable knowledge of IR.

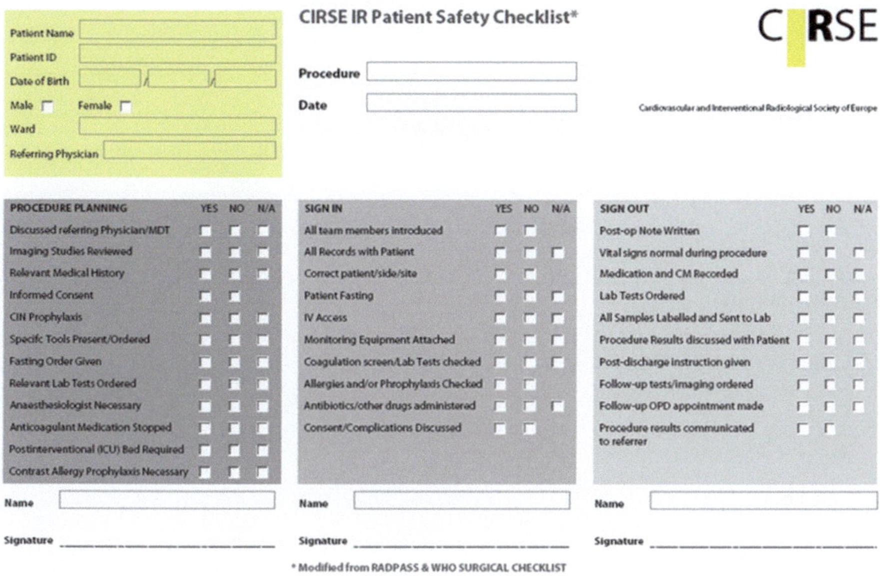
CIRSE IR Patient Safety Checklist*

CIRSE

Cardiovascular and Interventional Radiological Society of Europe

Patient Name
Patient ID
Date of Birth / /
Male Female
Ward
Referring Physician

Procedure
Date

PROCEDURE PLANNING	YES	NO	N/A
Discussed referring Physician/MDT	☐	☐	☐
Imaging Studies Reviewed	☐	☐	☐
Relevant Medical History	☐	☐	☐
Informed Consent	☐	☐	
CIN Prophylaxis	☐	☐	☐
Specific Tools Present/Ordered	☐	☐	☐
Fasting Order Given	☐	☐	☐
Relevant Lab Tests Ordered	☐	☐	☐
Anaesthesiologist Necessary	☐	☐	☐
Anticoagulant Medication Stopped	☐	☐	☐
Postinterventional (ICU) Bed Required	☐	☐	☐
Contrast Allergy Prophylaxis Necessary	☐	☐	☐

SIGN IN	YES	NO	N/A
All team members introduced	☐	☐	
All Records with Patient	☐	☐	☐
Correct patient/side/site	☐	☐	
Patient Fasting	☐	☐	☐
IV Access	☐	☐	☐
Monitoring Equipment Attached	☐	☐	☐
Coagulation screen/Lab Tests checked	☐	☐	☐
Allergies and/or Phrophylaxis Checked	☐	☐	
Antibiotics/other drugs administered	☐	☐	☐
Consent/Complications Discussed	☐	☐	

SIGN OUT	YES	NO	N/A
Post-op Note Written	☐	☐	
Vital signs normal during procedure	☐	☐	☐
Medication and CM Recorded	☐	☐	☐
Lab Tests Ordered	☐	☐	☐
All Samples Labelled and Sent to Lab	☐	☐	☐
Procedure Results discussed with Patient	☐	☐	☐
Post-discharge instruction given	☐	☐	☐
Follow-up tests/imaging ordered	☐	☐	☐
Follow-up OPD appointment made	☐	☐	☐
Procedure results communicated to referrer	☐	☐	

Name
Signature

Name
Signature

Name
Signature

* Modified from RADPASS & WHO SURGICAL CHECKLIST

Fig. 1.1 Typical patient safety checklist used in IR which includes a pre-procedure checklist, time out and post procedure checklist

- Routine blood investigations such as a full blood count, renal profile and a coagulation screen are usually required for most procedures.
- Occasionally and subject to local guidelines, blood investigations may not be required for some simple procedures such as superficial biopsies or venous procedures where haemostasis is easily achieved by local compression.
- The awareness of iodinated contrast material (CM) allergy is crucial before any proposed procedure where CM is used (endovascular procedures).
- A safety checklist (Fig. 1.1) has been developed and is now in routine use to ensure patient safety.

1.4 IR Practice

- IRs work in Interventional suites or 'angiographic laboratories' with the support of dedicated specialist nursing staff and radiographers or technologists (Fig. 1.2).
- These procedure suites are designed like operating theatres and most contemporary rooms have a clean air designation to improve procedure sterility.
- Many IRs also now lead a clinical service where they see patients in outpatient clinics, admit patients for many procedures and perform ward rounds on patients post-procedure. Collaboration and teamwork with referring clinicians and disciplines are essential.

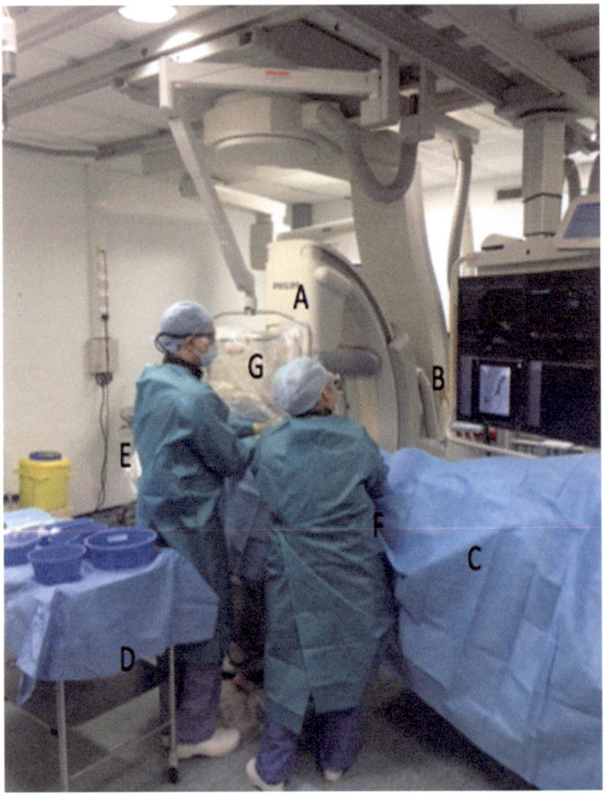

Fig. 1.2 Example of a percutaneous nephrostomy procedure being performed in an Interventional Radiology suite. *A* C-arm, *B* Monitor displaying live images, *C* Bed/ Patient, *D* Sterile trolley and IR equipment, *E* Interventional Radiologist, *F* Scrub Nurse, *G* Radiation protection screen

Key Points

- IR is a relatively new minimally invasive, image-guided specialty that has grown from Radiology.
- IR is often termed "Pinhole Surgery"
- IR is mandatory for modern healthcare delivery.
- IRs train in diagnostic and interventional radiology with some years of clinical practice also desirable.

Suggested Reading

1. European Board of Interventional Radiology. www.cirse.org.
2. IR curriculum and syllabus. www.cirse.org.
3. Patient safety checklist. www.cirse.org.

Principles, Signs and Symptoms of Peripheral Vascular Disease

2

Mark Sheehan, Hong Kuan Kok, and Michael Lee

2.1 Introduction

- Peripheral arterial disease (PAD) includes a group of conditions of different aetiologies which can affect the vessels of the upper and lower limb. PAD is most commonly used to describe atherosclerotic disease of the lower extremity arteries.
- PAD can be divided into acute and chronic presentations; the principal pathology being a compromised supply of oxygenated blood to the extremities leading to tissue ischaemia and necrosis if severe.

2.2 Risk Factors

- Smoking
- Hyperlipidemia
- Hypertension
- Age
- Diabetes Mellitus
- Male
- Family history
- Homocysteinemia

M. Sheehan • H.K. Kok • M. Lee (✉)
Department of Radiology, Beaumont Hospital and Royal College of Surgeons in Ireland, Dublin, Ireland
e-mail: marksheehan@rcsi.ie

H.K. Kok et al. (eds.), *Interventional Radiology for Medical Students*,
DOI 10.1007/978-3-319-53853-2_2

2.3 Chronic Lower Limb PAD

2.3.1 Symptoms

- The symptoms of PAD depend on the extent of arterial stenosis or occlusion and the presence or absence of collateral supply to the ischaemic limb.
- PAD is often classified into three categories, each indicating progressively more severe disease – intermittent claudication, rest pain and critical limb ischaemia.
- The Rutherford and Fontaine classifications are used to grade the symptoms of PAD:

Rutherford		Fontaine	
Stage	Clinical	Stage	Clinical
0	Asymptomatic	I	Asymptomatic
1	Mild claudication	IIa	Mild claudication
2	Moderate claudication	IIb	Moderate to Severe claudication
3	Severe claudication	III	Ischaemic rest pain
4	Ischaemic rest pain	IV	Ulceration or gangrene
5	Minor tissue loss		
6	Ulceration or gangrene		

2.3.1.1 Intermittent Claudication (IC)

- Defined as cramping muscular pain that develops on physical exertion and is relieved by rest. This pain typically occurs because there is an imbalance between the arterial supply and the metabolic demands of the muscles in the lower limb. The distance walked to onset of symptoms is quite consistent in each individual and is referred to as the claudication distance.
- Age adjusted prevalence of 12%, 20% of those presenting are over 70 years.
- 25% deteriorate – 7–9% in the first year and 2–3% thereafter
- Amputation rate is 1–3.3% over a 3 year period
- 5, 10, 15 year mortality rates are 30%, 50% and 70% respectively

2.3.1.2 Rest Pain

- Severe pain that typically affects the toes and forefoot without exertion (Rutherford 4 or Fontaine III). Symptoms often occur at night or when patient is at rest with the limbs elevated due to reduced gravity perfusion.
- Patients often report relief of pain by standing or when the leg is positioned over the edge of the bed. This is related to the gravitational effects of dependence on limb blood pressure.

2.3.1.3 Critical Limb Ischaemia (CLI)

- CLI is defined as severe arterial compromise in patients with peripheral arterial disease, often resulting in tissue loss. It includes severe rest pain, limb ulcers or gangrene (Rutherford 4–6 or Fontaine III–IV).

- There is a 20% mortality at 1 year and continues at the same rate. Mortality at 12 months is worse than many cancers.
- High risk of amputation with limb and mobility loss.
- Also associated with a high risk of cardiovascular events including myocardial infarction and death.

2.4 Clinical Signs

- Inspection:
  - Hair loss
  - Dystrophic skin and nail changes
  - Pallor
  - Arterial ulcers – Punched out, painful, deep, pressure points
  - Gangrene
  - Previous amputation
- Palpation (comparing both sides):
  - Cool peripheries
  - Reduced capillary refill time
  - Reduced or absent peripheral pulses: femoral, popliteal, dorsalis pedis and posterior tibial pulses
  - Blood pressure measurement
- Auscultation
  - Arterial bruits over the aorta, femoral, carotid arteries
- Special tests:
  - Buerger's test: Straight leg lift causing pallor in the foot and toes of a patient with PAD lying in the supine position. The angle when the signs are observed is known as Buerger's angle. Reactive hyperaemia is seen when the limb has been positioned dependently off the edge of the bed.

2.5 Investigations

- **Ankle-Brachial Index (ABI)**: This is a non-invasive measurement of the ratio of systolic blood pressure in the lower limb compared to that of the upper limb. Interpretation of ABI results is as follows:
  - Ratio of >1.2 – Associated with calcified non compressible arteries such as those occurring in patients with diabetes mellitus.
  - Ratio of 0.9–1.2 – Normal
  - Ratio of 0.4–0.9 – Mild to moderate PAD
  - Ratio < 0.4 – Severe PAD, usually associated with tissue loss
- **Toe Pressures**: This is another non-invasive measure of arterial insufficiency. It is particularly useful in diabetic patients with calcified non compressible vessels

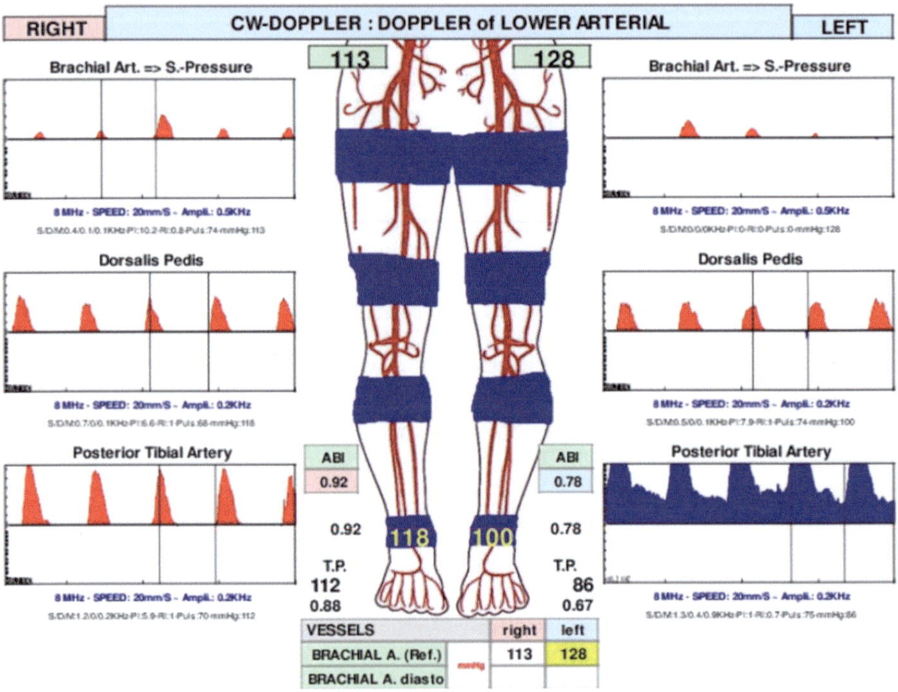

Fig. 2.1 Example of a report from the non-invasive Vascular Laboratory including Doppler measurements of arterial flow in the upper and lower limb arteries as well as ankle-brachial index (ABI) and toe pressure (TP) measurements in a patient with mild left lower extremity PAD (ABI 0.78 and Toe pressure of 86 mmHg)

and gives a more accurate representation of the arterial compromise in comparison to ABI measurements.

- Toe pressures <30 mmHg suggests severe PAD.
- A toe-brachial index (TBI) can also be calculated and interpreted in a similar manner to ABI (Fig. 2.1).
- **Duplex Ultrasound**: This is a non-invasive imaging study which combines the anatomic assessment of a blood vessel using ultrasound with the ability to assess blood flow using the Doppler technique.
- The extent and impact of a stenotic lesion on the flow of blood within a vessel can be accurately assessed.
- Duplex ultrasound does not involve ionising radiation and is a useful tool for both the diagnosis and follow-up of PAD.
- Disadvantages of duplex ultrasound include operator variability and a relatively long exam time (30–60 min) (Fig. 2.2).
- **CT Angiography (CTA)**: Non-invasive angiographic imaging of the aorta, visceral and peripheral arteries without the need for arterial catheterisation.

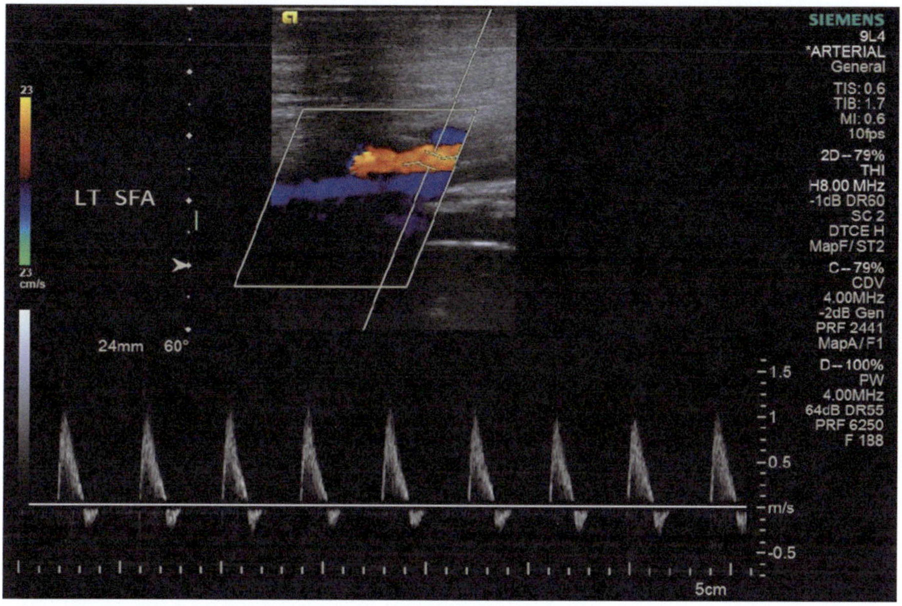

Fig. 2.2 Duplex ultrasound of the left superficial femoral artery demonstrating normal triphasic flow in the artery *(arrow)* consistent with patency

- Iodine-based contrast media is injected through a peripheral intravenous cannula followed by acquisition of high-resolution images with the contrast opacification timed to the arterial phase using a multidetector CT scanner.
- Modern CT scanners allow images to be reconstructed in multiple planes such as the coronal, sagittal or oblique planes to aid interpretation. Volumetric 3D reconstructions can be performed to aid pre-procedural planning.
- The advantages of CTA is the rapid acquisition of high-resolution images (seconds) and its non-invasive nature.
- Disadvantages include exposure to ionising radiation, risk of contrast induced nephropathy in patients with chronic renal impairment and reduced accuracy in the assessment of heavily calcified arteries due to 'blooming' artifacts (stenosis and occlusions may be overestimated) (Fig. 2.3).
- **Magnetic resonance angiogram (MRA)**: Non-invasive imaging technique, which is similar to CTA but does not involve ionising radiation and is therefore safer.
- Image acquisition generally involves administration of a gadolinium-based contrast agent through a peripheral intravenous cannula followed by imaging in an MRI scanner, consisting of a superconducting magnet (commonly at 1.5 or 3.0 Tesla field strength) and radiofrequency coils to obtain high-resolution images.
- However, MRA is contraindicated in patients with certain cardiac pacemakers, loose metal within or on the body and certain intracranial clips. Image quality is

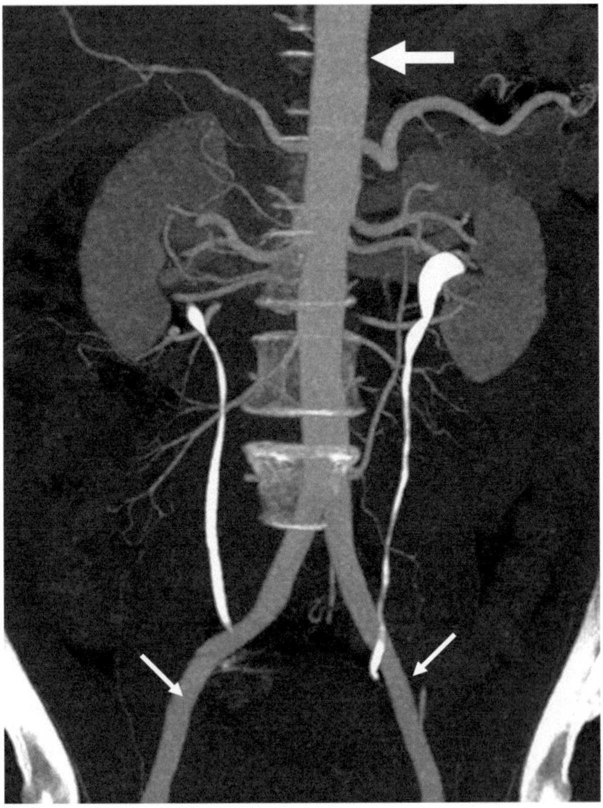

Fig. 2.3 Coronal CT angiogram reconstruction showing the abdominal aorta (*large arrow*), visceral branches and common iliac arteries (*small arrows*). Excreted iodinated contrast material is also present in the kidneys and ureters

also limited by metal implants such as knee or hip prosthesis and metallic stents due to distortion of the magnetic field.

- Advantages of MRA include better accuracy in imaging heavily calcified vessels, especially the infrapopliteal arteries and avoidance of ionising radiation.
- Disadvantages include a long scanning time (45–60 min) compared to CTA (seconds) and potential for patient claustrophobia due to the narrow bore of the MRI scanner. Gadolinium contrast agents may also cause nephrogenic systemic fibrosis in patients with severe renal impairment (Fig. 2.4).
- **Invasive Angiography**: Invasive angiography involves imaging the vascular system using a fluoroscopic x-ray machine and the injection of contrast material (usually iodine-based) directly into the vessel of interest following percutaneous access into the arterial system.
- Angiography provides information on the dynamic flow of blood as well as better spatial and temporal resolution than non-invasive imaging techniques such as

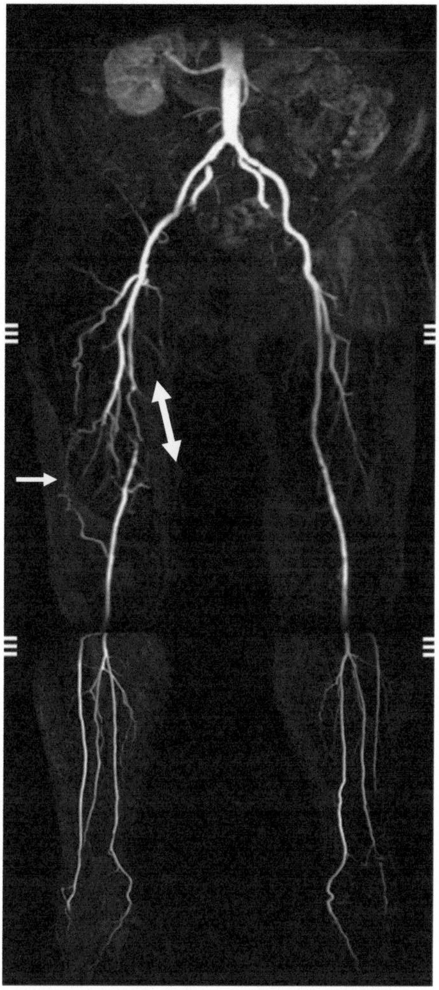

Fig. 2.4 MR angiogram of the peripheral arterial system following administration of a gadolinium-based contrast agent through a peripheral IV cannula. This example shows a segment of occlusion in the right superficial femoral artery (*long arrow*) but normal vessels below the level of occlusion. Smaller collateral vessels have developed to redirect flow beyond the occlusion (*short arrow*)

CTA or MRA. Images can be digitally subtracted (DSA) to remove structures such as bone and soft tissue to allow highly accurate vascular imaging. Angiography also provides superior assessment of small and heavily calcified vessels such as the infrapopliteal arteries.

- Disadvantages include the invasive nature of the procedure and it is therefore performed mostly prior to further treatment such as angioplasty and the risk of contrast induced nephropathy when large amounts of iodinated contrast material is administered. This will be discussed in further chapters (Fig. 2.5).

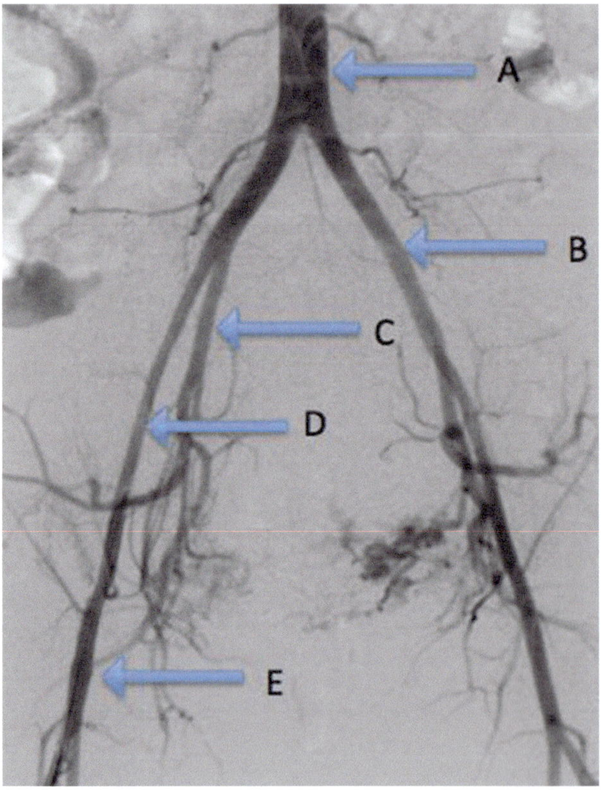

Fig. 2.5 Catheter digital subtraction angiogram (DSA) of the pelvis showing the (*A*) distal abdominal aorta, (*B*) left common iliac artery, (*C*) right internal and (*D*) external iliac artery (*C*), and the right common femoral artery (*E*)

2.6 Management

The management of patients with PAD is made on an individual basis following a consensus decision made at a Multi-disciplinary team meeting and depends on a wide variety of factors including patient symptoms, patient wishes and lesion anatomy.

- **Conservative**:
  - Risk factor modification: Optimal control of risk factors such as smoking cessation, hypertension, glycaemia in diabetics and weight loss.
  - Exercise therapy: In many claudicants, supervised exercise therpapy can increase claudication distance by promoting collateralisation of vessels.
  - Pharmacological: Statins, phosphodiesterase inhibitors (e.g. pentoxifyline and cilostazol).
- **Endovascular**:
  - Percutaneous angioplasty and stenting
    See following chapter.

- **Surgery**:
  - Surgical bypass
    - The segment of stenosis or occlusion is "bypassed" with a venous or synthethic graft. Venous grafts are preferred due to improved patency and lower risk of infection.
    - Examples include – Femoral to popliteal ('fem-pop') and femoral to distal bypass procedures.
    - Ilio-femoral bypass procedures are performed in younger patients with extensive iliac occlusions. Good long term patency is observed but with a cost in terms of an 8% operative mortality and 15% serious morbidity.
    - An "endovascular first" strategy is now increasingly used in PAD patients
  - Amputation
    - Generally reserved as a last resort for CLI with severe gangrene or tissue loss, often with unmanageable local infection.

2.7 Acute Limb Ischaemia

- Patients with acute limb ischaemia present with acute onset symptoms which include **p**ain, **p**allor, **p**aresthesia, **p**ulselessness, **p**aralysis and **p**erishingly cold limb (the six P's).
- The aetiology of acute ischaemia is usually secondary to embolisation, thrombus formation or trauma (such as dissection) to the arteries.
- Embolisation is typically from a cardiac source such as thrombus in the left atrial appendage in patients with atrial fibrillation, a left ventricular mural thrombus following myocardial infarction or as a complication following a vascular procedure.
- Management:
  - Systemic anticoagulation: If the cause is secondary to thromboembolic pathology, systemic anticoagulation with heparin should be commenced provided that there are no contraindications.
  - Surgical embolectomy using a Fogarty balloon catheter, particularly if the extremity is threatened or if a large burden of thrombus is present.
  - Catheter directed thrombolysis: An intraarterial infusion catheter can be positioned within the thrombus to allow direct delivery of thrombolytic agents such as tissue plasminogen activator resulting in lysis of the thrombus. Generally, the more acute the presentation, the more successful the result from thrombolysis.

Key Points

- In the clinical history, it is important to identify cardiovascular risk factors, differentiating the patterns of pain and deciding whether the patient has intermittent claudication, rest pain or CLI.
- Clinical examination is based on inspection, palpation, auscultation and the use of Buerger's test.

- Investigations include non-invasive measurement of ABI or toe pressures as well as imaging tests such as Duplex ultrasound, CTA or MRA which shows the level and severity of disease and guides further management.
- Aggressive risk factor modification is required for all patients including smoking cessation and appropriate medical therapy.
- For claudicants, supervised exercise therapy can be attempted in patients with relatively long claudication distances (>100 m). Short distance claudicants or those with occlusive iliac disease can be considered for further endovascular or surgical management following multidisciplinary consensus.
- For patients with critical limb ischemia, endovascular or surgical intervention is required to restore in-line blood flow to the foot. This allows ulcers to heal and any gangrene to demarcate. Revascularisation also helps limit the extent of amputation (e.g. toe or transmetatarsal) and aids recovery.

Vascular Access and Equipment for Endovascular Interventions

3

Gareth Kiernan and Hong Kuan Kok

3.1 Introduction

- The most fundamental aspect of endovascular interventional radiology is securing vascular access in a safe and effective manner.
- Once this has been achieved, a wide variety and steadily expanding range of equipment can be delivered as needed including introducer sheaths, guidewires, catheters, angioplasty balloons, stents, embolisation materials and finally, access site closure devices to name but a few.

3.2 Vascular Access

- Vascular access is generally achieved using a combination of manual palpation of the vessel of interest based on anatomical landmarks or increasingly through the assistance of image guidance, predominantly using ultrasound or fluoroscopy.
- Either the arterial or venous circulation can be accessed depending on the required procedure.

G. Kiernan
Department of Radiology, Beaumont Hospital, Dublin, Ireland
e-mail: gary_kiernan@hotmail.com

H.K. Kok (✉)
Department of Radiology, Beaumont Hospital and Royal College of Surgeons in Ireland, Dublin, Ireland

H.K. Kok et al. (eds.), *Interventional Radiology for Medical Students*,
DOI 10.1007/978-3-319-53853-2_3

- Common arterial puncture sites include the common femoral, brachial, popliteal, pedal and radial arteries with location determined by the intervention to be performed. Arterial puncture sites should ideally be performed adjacent to a bony structure to allow adequate compression for haemostasis.
- Common venous puncture sites include the common femoral, internal jugular, subclavian and peripheral veins of the upper arm (basilic, cephalic or brachial).

3.3 Seldinger Technique for Vascular Access

- The most common vascular access technique is the Seldinger technique named after the Swedish radiologist, Dr. Sven-Ivar Seldinger. Current vascular access techniques involve slight variations of the Seldinger method, known as the 'modified' Seldinger technique.
- Following localisation of the vessel to be accessed, a vascular access needle which has a hollow core is advanced until bleed back is achieved (Fig. 3.1a).
- A guidewire is then placed through the needle core into the vessel (Fig. 3.1b).

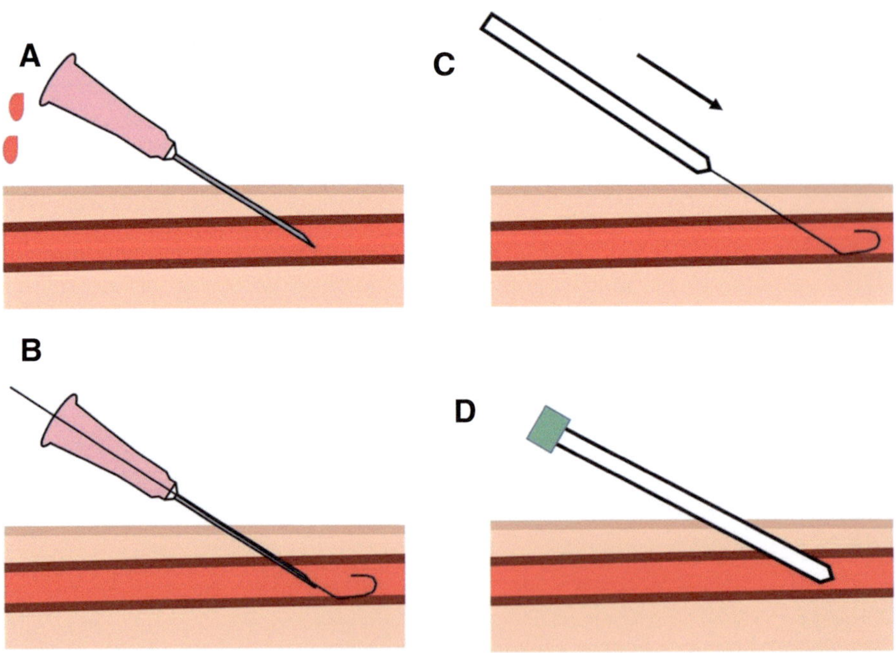

Fig. 3.1 Seldinger technique for vascular access. A hollow needle is used to puncture the anterior wall of the artery or vein (**a**). Through this needle, a J-shaped guidewire is inserted into the artery or vein and the needle removed while holding firm pressure on the access point (**b**). An introducer sheath is then inserted over the guidewire into the artery or vein (**c**). Through this sheath, various catheters, balloons or stents can be placed depending on the goal of treatment (**d**)

- The needle is then removed over the guidewire and an introducer sheath or catheter is inserted into the vessel over the guidewire (Fig. 3.1c).
- Vascular access is thus secured and all other endovascular equipment that is needed for a given procedure can be inserted into the vessel via a sheath or catheter (Fig. 3.1d).

3.4 Guidewires

- Guidewires are a key element in both vascular and non-vascular interventional procedures including hepatobiliary, gastrointestinal and urological procedures.
- Guidewires generally consist of a soft atraumatic tip to minimise injury to the vessel wall during advancement. Guidewire length is measured in centimeters and the diameter is measured in inches (e.g. 0.014, 0.018 and 0.035 inch).
- Guidewires are available in different levels of stiffness depending on the clinical need, ranging from soft general purpose wires (e.g. Bentson) to very stiff wires used in aortic interventions (e.g. Lunderquist).
- They can be further classified into steerable and non-steerable guidewires. Non-steerable wires act as a support system that enable catheters and other devices to be 'guided' into position. Steerable guidewires are used to navigate tortuous, diseased and narrowed vasculature or to help select specific vessels. These often have a shaped tip or a tip that can be shaped by the operator.
- Most guidewires are composed of a stainless steel or nitinol (nickel-titanium) core and may contain a polymer coating which decreases friction and allows easier advancement.
- More specialised guidewires may be coated in specific materials such as a hydrophilic material which becomes very slippery when wet and can navigate highly tortuous vessels and stenoses.

3.5 Catheters

- Catheters are hollow flexible tubes predominantly composed of polymer and are available in a wide variety of shapes and sizes. They are generally advanced over guidewires and can also be coated in specific materials including hydrophilic substances.
- Catheter length is measured in centimeters however the external diameter is measured in French (Fr) size, which when divided by three approximates the external diameter in millimeters. For example, a 6 French catheter size corresponds to external diameter of approximately 2 mm.
- Catheters can be broadly classified into selective and non-selective types. Selective catheters have specially shaped tips and a single end-hole to allow easier access to particular vessels or side branches. There are a wide selection of such catheters commercially available and most interventional suites will have a selection of commonly used shapes.

- Specially designed catheters include microcatheters which are generally under 3 French in size, can be passed through 5 or 6 Fr catheters and are used in navigating through very small or tortuous vessels.
- Non-selective catheters are used in larger vessels for diagnostic angiography and contain multiple side-holes in addition to an end-hole. Examples include the pigtail catheter, which is used in larger vessels. The pigtail shape prevents it from inadvertently entering smaller vessels where contrast injection at a high rate can result in vascular injury.
- In vascular interventions, catheters are used for angiography and also as delivery systems for therapeutic devices such as embolisation materials or drugs.

3.6 Sheaths

- Any procedure may involve the use of several devices including multiple guidewires and catheters. To allow for multiple device exchanges, an introducer sheath is generally inserted into the vessel at the start of the procedure.
- This consists of a hollow tube attached to a hemostatic valve which prevents back bleeding and blood loss during a procedure. A sheath may also have a side port for flushing with saline or contrast (Fig. 3.2).
- Sheath sizes are also measured using the French size but this refers to the inner diameter of the sheath tubing as opposed to the external diameter as in the case of catheters. This is because a 5 French sheath (inner diameter) for example, has to be able to accommodate a 5 French catheter (outer diameter).

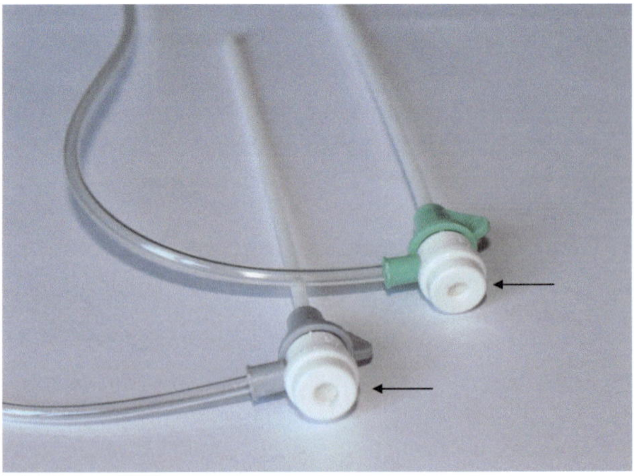

Fig. 3.2 Introducer sheaths with haemostatic valves (*arrows*) and side ports for flushing

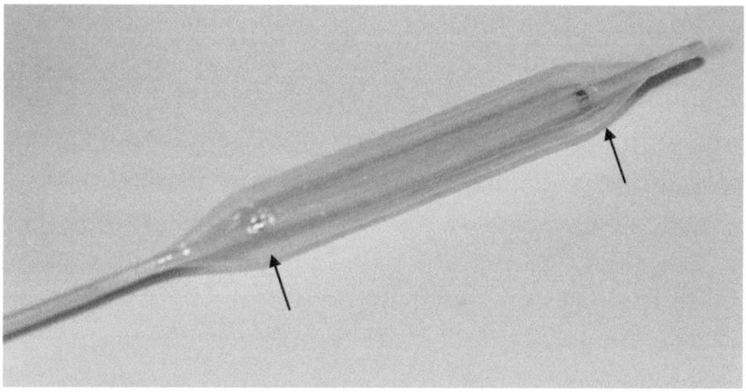

Fig. 3.3 Angioplasty balloon following inflation. Radiopaque marker bands (*arrows*) on the balloon allow visualisation of the balloon position using fluoroscopy

3.7 Angioplasty Balloons

- Percutaneous transluminal angioplasty (PTA) involves using an angioplasty balloon to dilate a vascular stenosis or occlusion (Fig. 3.3).
- Angioplasty balloons are mounted on a catheter delivery system which is introduced into the vessel over a guidewire in the same way as a standard angiography catheter.
- The angioplasty balloon catheter is advanced to the segment of vessel to be treated using fluoroscopic guidance. Subsequently, the balloon is inflated with a syringe or inflation device using dilute iodinated contrast material.
- Angioplasty balloons come in a variety of sizes and lengths and are measured in millimeters (e.g. 6 mm diameter by 80 mm length) are sized according to the vessel that requires treatment.
- The treatment of vascular stenoses or occlusions may involve PTA alone or PTA followed by stenting to maintain vascular patency.
- Specialised angioplasty balloons may be coated with antiproliferative drugs such as paclitaxel (drug-coated balloon) to reduce neointimal hyperplasia and therefore, increase the long-term durability of PTA. Other angioplasty balloon types include high-pressure and cutting balloons which are used to treat heavily fibrotic or very resistant lesions to conventional PTA.

3.8 Metal Stents

- Metal stents were originally introduced to address the limitations of angioplasty, most notably elastic recoil, restenosis or dissection following PTA.
- Elastic recoil involves 'collapse' of a vessel after PTA, usually due to arterial wall calcification or because of hard, fibrotic stenoses. Dissection occurs commonly during PTA due to detachment of the intimal layer from the media and may be flow limiting when large. Stents act as a scaffold to maintain patency in these situations.

- Stents can be broadly categorised into balloon expandable or self-expandable stents and are sized in the same way as angioplasty balloons (e.g. 8 mm diameter and 100 mm length stent). Regardless of the stent type, all stents are delivered over a guidewire.
- Balloon expandable stents are mounted onto an angioplasty balloon catheter and are deployed in situ when the balloon is inflated. They are usually made of stainless steel or a cobalt-chromium alloy.
- Self-expanding stents are delivered through a co-axial delivery catheter system. The stent itself is collapsed and contained within the delivery system. During deployment, the outer sheath of this catheter is retracted and the constrained stent expands into its natural shape. These stents are usually made of a nickel-titanium alloy (nitinol) which has the unique property of expanding back to its natural shape and has high flexibility.
- Some stents are coated with an anti-proliferative agent such as paclitaxel and are known as drug-eluting stents. The antiproliferative drug reduces neointimal hyperplasia which in turn, reduces restenosis rates. In recent years, there has been significant interest in bioresorbable stents which essentially dissolve after a certain time period.
- Some metal stents have a polymer covering and are called covered stents. These are used to treat aneurysms (including aortic), to seal a bleeding artery and to prevent neointimal hyperplasia (Fig. 3.4).

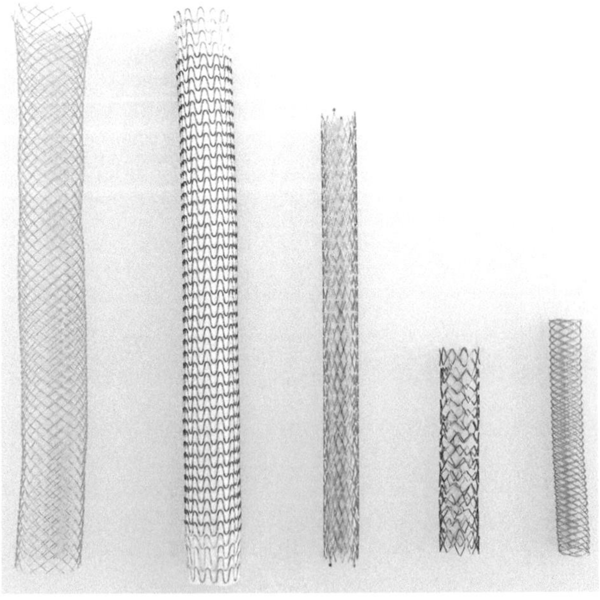

Fig. 3.4 Metallic vascular stents of varying size, length and design characteristics

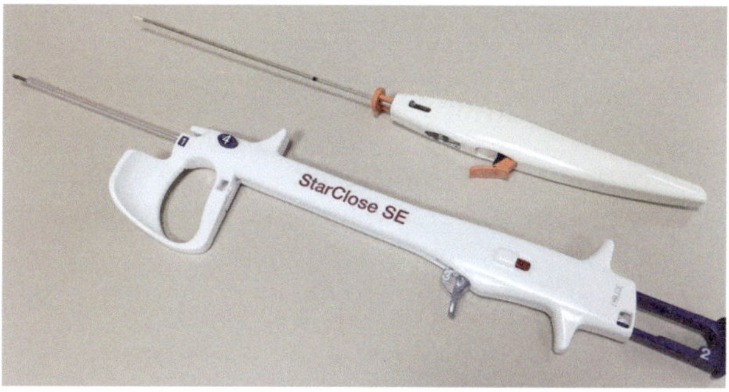

Fig. 3.5 Example of vascular closure devices Cordis Exoseal (*above*) and Abbott StarClose SE (*below*)

3.9 Access Site Closure and After Care

- Following completion of an interventional procedure, the sheath is withdrawn from the artery and haemostasis is achieved through manual pressure over the puncture site for approximately 10–30 min, depending on the size of the sheath and the use of intraprocedural anticoagulation.
- In addition, a selection of vascular closure devices are available as an alterative to prolonged manual compression. Examples include the AngioSeal (Terumo), Perclose (Abbott), Starclose (Abbott) and ExoSeal (Cordis) devices. Vascular closure devices can reduce time to haemostasis and ambulation, medical resources input and expedite hospital discharge (Fig. 3.5).
- However, the use of these devices can also introduce device specific complications such as deployment problems and infection.
- Following femoral arterial access, bedrest for 4–6 h is required followed by gradual ambulation. The access site should be carefully observed for the development of a haematoma or pseudoaneurysm and distal pulses should be examined.
- Vital signs including pulse and blood pressure measurements should be recorded regularly to detect evidence of occult blood loss such as retroperitoneal haemorrhage.

3.10 Complications

Complications may be divided into local-access site, procedural and systemic complications:

Access site complications (overall 2.3–33%):

- Haematoma (local 1–10% and retroperitoneal <1%)
- Pseudoaneurysm (0.2–2%)
- Acute occlusion/dissection (<1%)

- Distal embolisation (1.6–2.4%)
- Arteriovenous fistula (<1%)
- Infection (very rare)

Procedure related complications:
Depends on specific procedure and will be discussed in corresponding chapters but include:

- Arterial dissection (variable, technique dependent)
- Arterial rupture (variable, technique dependent)
- Arterial occlusion (<1%)
- Arteriovenous fistula (<1%)
- Device specific complications (variable, device dependent)
- Limb loss (0.6–2.2%) and death (0–1%)

Systemic complications:

- Atheromatous/cholesterol embolisation to distal extremities (1.6–2.4%)
- Stroke – neurovascular procedures and interventions involving the aortic arch (variable, procedure dependent)
- Contrast reaction (<0.1%)
- Contrast induced nephropathy (2–20%)
- Complications of anticoagulation or thrombolysis including major bleeding (2.9–13.3% depending on thrombolytic agent and dose)

Key Points

- The most fundamental aspect of vascular interventional radiology is obtaining and securing vascular access in a safe and effective manner, most commonly using the Seldinger technique.
- A variety of vascular tools are available ranging from introducer sheaths, catheters and guidewires to angioplasty balloons and stents.
- Complications of endovascular interventions include local access site, procedural and systemic complications. Meticulous aftercare is an important part of patient management.

Further Reading

1. Katsanos K, Tepe G, Tsetis D, Fanelli F. Standards of practice for superficial femoral and popliteal artery angioplasty and stenting. Cardiovasc Intervent Radiol 2014;37:592–603.
2. Karnabatidis D, Spiliopoulos S, Tsetis D, Siablis D. Quality improvement guidelines for percutaneous catheter-directed intra-arterial thrombolysis and mechanical Thrombectomy for acute lower-limb ischemia. Cardiovasc Intervent Radiol 2011;34:1123–1136.

Endovascular Treatment of Peripheral Arterial Disease

4

Hong Kuan Kok

4.1 Introduction

- Peripheral arterial disease (PAD) is a manifestation of systemic atherosclerosis, most commonly affecting the arterial supply of the lower limbs. Clinical presentation can range from asymptomatic lesions to intermittent claudication and tissue necrosis which may be complicated by superimposed infection (so called "wet gangrene").
- Patients with PAD can also present acutely with symptoms secondary to thromboembolism or vascular trauma in which urgent intervention is required. Most patients will undergo a range of investigations including ankle-brachial index measurements and imaging with Duplex ultrasound or CT/MR angiography to assess the extent and severity of disease.
- Imaging of PAD can reveal lesions ranging from a single stenosis to complex multifocal stenoses or long chronic total occlusions which will influence management and the technical approach adapated.
- Management of PAD is centered around comprehensive management of cardiovascular risk factors including smoking cessation, regular exercise and optimal medical therapy for hypertension, dyslipidaemia and diabetes.
- Patients who do not respond to conservative therapy may require further intervention either in the form of surgical bypass procedures or increasingly, minimally invasive endovascular therapy such as angioplasty and stenting.

H.K. Kok
Department of Radiology, Beaumont Hospital and Royal College of Surgeons in Ireland, Dublin, Ireland
e-mail: terrykok@gmail.com

H.K. Kok et al. (eds.), *Interventional Radiology for Medical Students*,
DOI 10.1007/978-3-319-53853-2_4

4.2 Indications

- Endovascular treatment of PAD is indicated in patients not adequately managed by conservative measures including severe intermittent claudication, critical limb ischaemia with rest pain, ulceration or gangrene. Mild to moderate claudication is usually managed conservatively with a supervised exercise therapy program.
- Treatment of acute lower limb ischaemia due to a variety of causes including arterial thromboembolism and trauma (dissection, rupture, occlusion).
- Procedures may be performed as a means of limb salvage in patients with tissue necrosis and infection with the aim of either avoiding surgical amputation or limiting the extent of amputation (i.e. avoiding major below or above knee amputations).

4.3 Contraindications

- Uncorrectable coagulopathy
- Medically unstable or critically ill patients in whom procedure benefit is outweighed by risk of complications
- Contraindication to antiplatelet or anticoagulation therapy
- Allergy to iodinated contrast agents – relative contraindication as carbon dioxide (CO_2) can be used as an alternative contrast agent
- Advanced renal impairment – relative contraindication as CO_2 can be used

4.4 Patient Preparation

- Discussion at a multidisciplinary meeting with comprehensive review of symptoms, signs, investigations and imaging with input from referring clinicians, vascular surgeons and interventional radiology.
- Can be performed as a day or short-stay procedure in selected patients.
- Fasting for 6 hours prior to the procedure.
- Confirm medical and surgical history paying attention to previous surgical bypass or endovascular interventions which may influence the procedure to be performed.
- Assess for any history of medication allergies and renal impairment which may preclude administration of iodinated contrast agents. These can be comprehensively assessed with a patient safety checklist as advocated by CIRSE (see Chap. 1).
- Intravenous access, ideally at least 18 gauge for IV fluid infusion, conscious sedation and resuscitation measures if necessary.
- Blood investigations including a contemporaneous full blood count, renal function tests and coagulation studies. Most operators would use a cut-off international normalised ratio (INR) of less than 1.5 and platelet count of greater than 50,000.
- Ensure appropriate medications are withheld prior to procedure following discussion with senior clinicians. In particular, anticoagulants will need adequate time for normalisation of coagulation status or reversal agents as appropriate depending on the urgency of the procedure. Many patients with PAD are on anticoagulation with warfarin or novel oral anticoagulants (e.g. rivaroxaban, dabigatran) for various indications which can increase procedural bleeding risk.

- Patients with PAD may also have chronic kidney disease of varying severity and consultation with an appropriate Nephrology service should be considered. Endovascular intervetions involve administration of iodinated contrast agents which are nephrotoxic in large volumes. Depending on local practice, patients may require prehydration with intravenous fluids (0.9% normal saline at 1 ml/kg/hr. for 24 h) and n-acetylcysteine (600 mg BID day before, day of and day after procedure).
- Insulin dependent diabetics may need a glucose-potassium-insulin (GKI) infusion while the intervention is being performed

4.5 Complications

Complications specific to the procedure generally include:

- Access site haematoma (1–10%) and pseudoaneurysm formation (0.2–2%).
- Retroperitoneal haemorrhage, which may require blood transfusion, embolisation or surgical intervention (<1%).
- Injury to treated vessel including dissection, perforation, rupture and distal embolisation (overall <3%). Risk of distal embolisation is higher in thrombolysis for acute ischaemia (3.8–24%).
- Major adverse event requiring emergency surgery (<3.5%).
- Major amputation (0.6–2.2%).
- Infection of implanted devices such as stents or stent-grafts (very rare).
- Allergic reaction to contrast agents (0.1%).
- Acute kidney injury secondary to contrast agents (2–20%).
- Mortality (<1%).

4.6 Medications

- Local anaesthesia to the vascular access site (e.g. lignocaine)
- Conscious sedation with short acting benzodiazepine and opioid analgesic
- Antiplatelet agents such as aspirin and clopidogrel
- Unfractionated heparin administered during the procedure
- Antibiotic prophylaxis is not indicated in most routine procedures. However, patients may already be on antibiotics for treatment of infected gangrene or osteomyelitis and this should continue during the periprocedural period. In addiition, if a synthetic vascular graft is going to be punctured to gain access, antibiotics are given.

4.7 Results

- Technical success for angioplasty and stenting are high, in excess of 90%.
- In general, primary patency rates of 70–80% at 1 year, 60–70% at 3 years and ~50% at 5 years can be expected following angioplasty and stenting in the femoral and popliteal arteries. These results are higher in the iliac arteries where primary patency rates of >80% at 3 years and >70% at 5 years are reported.
- Primary patency at 1 year following endovascular treatment is higher for stenting (>70%) when compared to angioplasty alone (between 50–60%) and even

higher with drug eluting stents (>85%) but this depends on the lesion morphology, calcification and length.

- Recently developed technologies including drug coated angioplasty balloons, drug eluting stents and braided nitinol stents show higher patency rates ranging from 80–90% but long term results are lacking.

4.8 Case Examples

Case 4.1

A 65 year-old man with worsening intermittent claudication in his left calf, now significantly limiting his lifestyle with a claudication distance of 50 meters. He underwent an MR angiogram of the lower limbs which showed a long 20 cm occlusion involving the left superficial femoral artery (SFA). His case was discussed at the vascular multidisciplinary conference and a consensus for endovascular treatment was made following discussion with the patient. As the vessel was completely occluded, a subintimal angioplasty technique was used (Figs. 4.1 and 4.2).

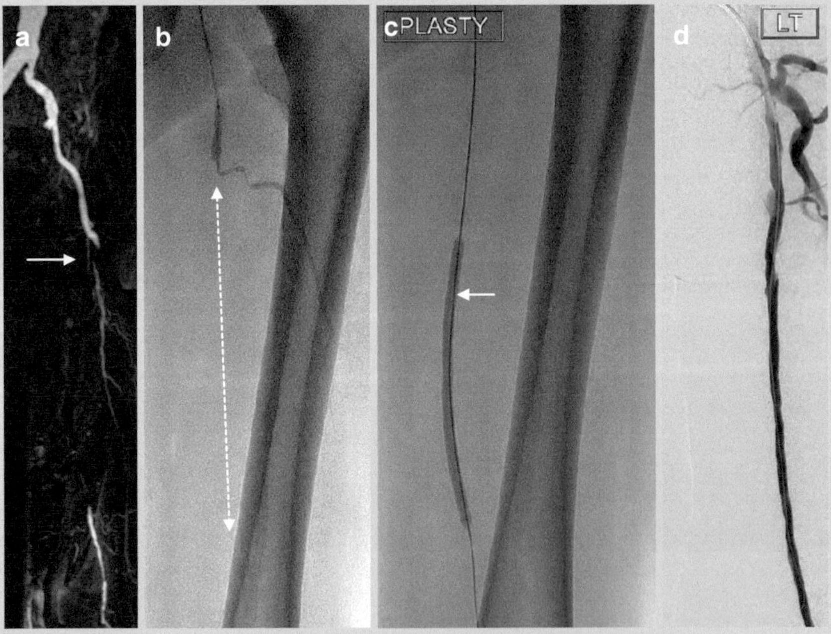

Fig. 4.1 (**a**) MR angiogram image showing occlusion of the left SFA (*arrow*). (**b**) Following an antegrade puncture of the left common femoral artery, a 6 French introducer sheath was placed and the occlusion was confirmed on angiography as shown by absence of contrast within the expected location of the SFA (*dotted line*). (**c**) Using a subintimal angioplasty technique, the occluded SFA was recanalised and angioplasty was performed with a balloon catheter (*arrow*). (**d**) Completion angiogram shows successful recanalisation of the SFA which is now opacified by contrast along its entire length. The patients symptoms resolved following this treatment and his medical therapy was optimised

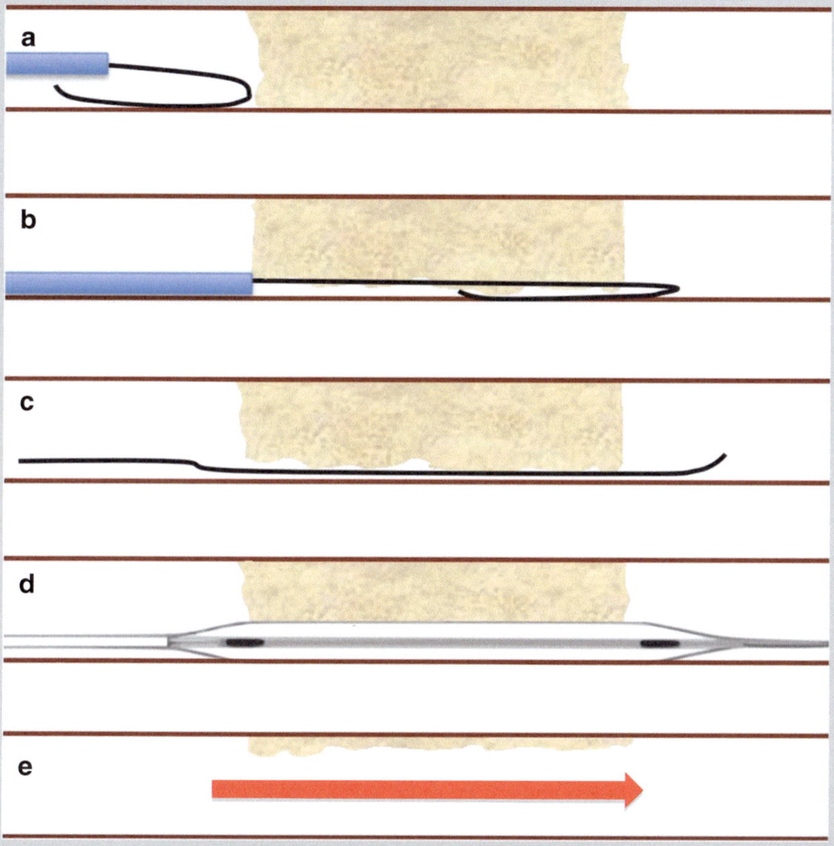

Fig. 4.2 Technique of subintimal angioplasty. (**a**) Using a combination of an angiographic catheter and an angled tip hydrophilic guidewire, a loop is formed at the level of the arterial occlusion to create a dissection between the intima and media of the artery. (**b**) The wire loop is advanced through the subintimal space beyond the occlusion and (**c**) re-entry into the true arterial lumen is achieved. (**d**) The catheter is exchanged for an appropriate size angioplasty balloon and subintimal angioplasty is performed to dilate the channel. (**e**) Final result following angioplasty with flow restored through the new subintimal channel

Case 4.2

An 80-year old female patient with multiple medical comorbidities including emphysema, coronary artery disease and ischaemic cardiomyopathy presents with severe rest pain in her left foot which keeps her awake at night. There was no evidence of ulceration or gangrene and her popliteal and distal pedal pulses were weak. A CT angiogram of her lower limbs was performed which showed a severe stenosis in the distal left SFA. Following discussion of treatment options at a multidisciplinary meeting and with the patient, endovascular treatment was chosen (Fig. 4.3).

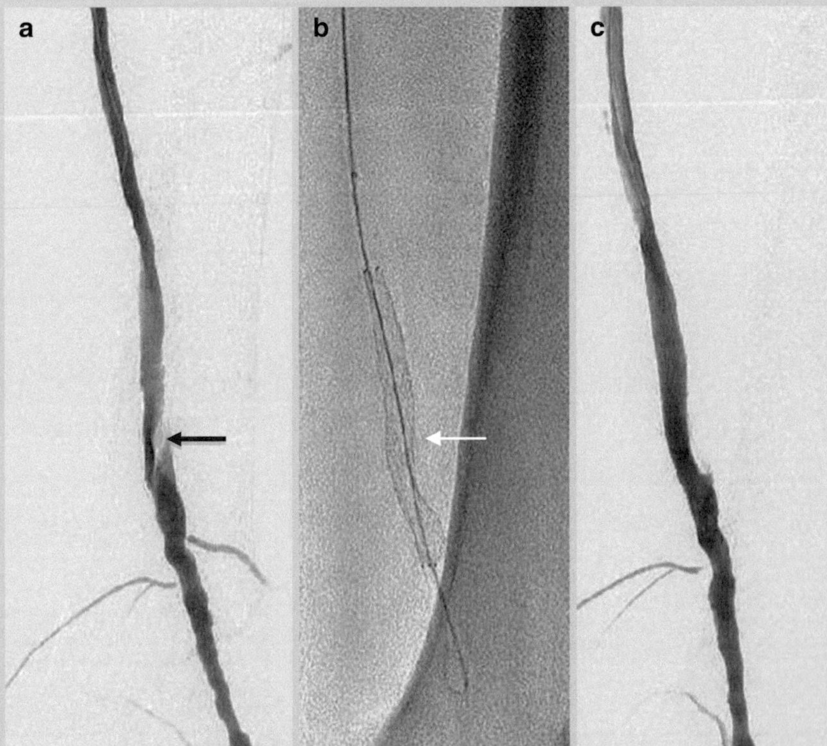

Fig. 4.3 (**a**) Left lower limb angiogram showed severe stenosis in the distal SFA at the level of the adductor hiatus. This was initially treated with angioplasty which resulted in a focal flow-limiting dissection (*arrow*). (**b**) Subsequently, a self-expanding stent was placed (*arrow*) and (**c**) the final angiographic result was improved. Her symptoms resolved following treatment and she remains on long-term antiplatelet therapy to maintain stent patency

4.9 Post-procedure Care and Review

- Bed rest for 4–6 h following the procedure with gradual mobilisation.
- Observation of vital signs and access site for local complications including haematoma and pseudoaneurysm formation. If this is suspected, further imaging should be performed, initially with a Duplex ultrasound of the access site.
- If the patients' vital signs deteriorate, bleeding from the groin into the retroperitoneum should be considered and manual presure applied to the groin during resuscitation.
- Examination of distal pulses and capillary refill.
- Commencement of appropriate medications such as antiplatelet therapy or a period of systemic anticoagulation depending on the individual case.
- Follow-up in the form of clinical assessment of symptoms and signs and/or imaging studies following intervention.

4.10 Discussion

- PAD is most commonly due to atherosclerosis and can affect any artery in the body. There is a predilection for involvement of the carotid (leading to TIA and stroke), coronary (angina and acute coronary syndromes) and peripheral lower limb arteries (intermittent claudication and critical limb ischaemia).
- In the lower limb, the iliac, femoral, popliteal and below knee tibial arteries are commonly involved. Atherosclerotic lesions in PAD often produce stenoses which can progress to total occlusions over time.
- Endovascular intervention for PAD involves a variety of techniques including balloon angioplasty and stenting. Other specialised techniques such as subintimal angioplasty, atherectomy, thrombolysis and thrombectomy may also be employed depending on characteristics of the lesion.
- Careful review of pre-procedural imaging will help the interventionalist plan the required techniques to perform the procedure effectively and safely.
- Most stenotic lesions can be treated using a luminal approach with conventional balloon angioplasty however chronic total occlusions often require a specialised technique called subintimal angioplasty, where a controlled dissection between the intima and media is formed across the occluded segment (Case 4.1). Importantly, these techniques do not preclude future surgical bypass.
- Occasionally, a suboptimal result may achieved with balloon angioplasty alone either because the lesion is resistant to angioplasty or because a complication such as dissection arises, requiring stenting to maintain vessel patency (Case 4.2).
- Newer techniques including the use of drug-coated angioplasty balloons, stents and bioabsorbable vascular scaffolds are under investigation with the promise of better patency rates however long-term clinical outcomes are awaited.

Key Points

- PAD is most commonly a manifestation of systemic atherosclerosis and requires aggressive reduction of cardiovascular risk factors and optimal medical therapy.
- Endovascular treatments for PAD are minimally invasive and effective in treating a variety of lesions in the iliac, femoral, popliteal and below knee tibial arteries.
- Patients with mild to moderate intermittent claudication should undergo supervised exercise therapy. Patients with severe claudication, rest pain and tissue loss in the form of ulcers or gangrene should be considered for endovascular treatment or surgical bypass if unsuccessful.
- Careful clinical and imaging assessment, multidisciplinary involvement and attention to pre and post-procedural care are essential.

Further Reading

1. Katsanos K, Tepe G, Tsetis D, Fanelli F. Standards of practice for superficial femoral and popliteal artery angioplasty and stenting. Cardiovasc Intervent Radiol 2014;37:592–603.
2. Rossi M, Iezzi R. Cardiovascular and interventional Society of Europe guidelines on endovascular treatment in aortoiliac arterial disease. Cardiovasc Intervent Radiol 2014;37:13–25.

Acute Embolisation Procedures 5

Hong Kuan Kok and Mark F. Given

5.1 Introduction and Embolisation Materials

- Embolisation is a minimally invasive technique used to occlude vascular supply to organs, tumours or vascular malformations. This often involves the precise delivery of embolic materials under imaging guidance with fluoroscopy, ultrasound or CT.
- The interventionalist has a choice of embolic materials to choose from depending on the clinical scenario and desired therapeutic outcome. These include specially designed devices such as metallic coils and vascular plugs, microparticles, gelatine sponges and liquid agents such as glue, thrombin or non-adhesive liquid embolics (ethylene vinyl alcohol copolymer) (Fig. 5.1).
- Acute embolisation procedures are performed in emergency situations such as in the trauma patient to control haemorrhage. This is often performed as an alternative or adjunct to more invasive surgical treatment.
- These procedures require close teamwork between interventional radiologists and many individuals of the trauma team including referring clinicians, trauma surgeons, anaesthetists, nurses and radiographers to deliver a safe and efficient service to the critically ill patient.

H.K. Kok (✉)
Department of Radiology, Beaumont Hospital and Royal College of Surgeons in Ireland, Dublin, Ireland
e-mail: terrykok@gmail.com

M.F. Given
Department of Radiology, Beaumont Hospital, Dublin, Ireland

H.K. Kok et al. (eds.), *Interventional Radiology for Medical Students*,
DOI 10.1007/978-3-319-53853-2_5

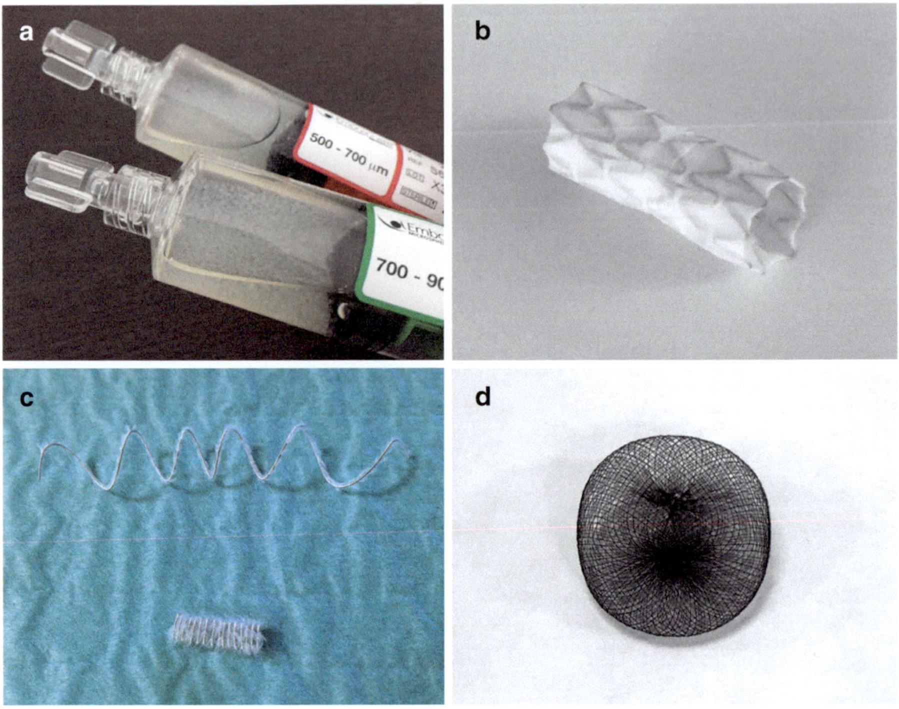

Fig. 5.1 Examples of embolisation materials available including (**a**) calibrated microparticles, (**b**) covered stent-grafts, (**c**) metallic coil and (**d**) vascular plug

5.2 Clinical Scenarios and Indications

5.2.1 Trauma and Visceral Injury

- Interventional radiology has a central role in the management of trauma patients, from providing rapid diagnosis through specialist imaging (ultrasound and CT) to interventional procedures.
- Bleeding from vascular (thoracic, abdominal and pelvic arterial branches) and visceral injuries (renal, liver, splenic injuries) can be managed through embolisation procedures in selected patients. In many cases, these procedures are life-saving and can avoid the morbidity of invasive surgery or can stabilise a critically ill patient for further definitive surgical treatment.

5.2.2 Gastrointestinal Tract Bleeding

- Acute upper or lower gastrointestinal tract bleeding can be treated with selective embolisation of bleeding vessels, particularly if other methods including endoscopy have been unsuccessful.
- Virtually any mesenteric vessel can be targeted and treated with embolisation. Commonly treated vessels include the gastroduodenal artery in upper gastrointestinal

bleeding and distal branches of the mesenteric arteries in lower gastrointestinal bleeding. The bleeding artery is selected as distally as possible to avoid precipitating ischemia to a particular segment of bowel and is typically embolised with metallic coils.

5.2.3 Haemoptysis

- Massive haemoptysis from bronchiectasis, cystic fibrosis, pulmonary tuberculosis and tumours can also be treated with embolisation.
- Most cases of large volume haemoptysis originate from hypertrophied or eroded bronchial or less commonly, intercostal arteries. These vessels can be embolised using microparticles.

5.2.4 Epistaxis

- Epistaxis is a common condition, usually arising from the anterior septal area (Little's area) and less commonly from the posterior nasal cavity.
- The vascular supply to the nasal septum is derived mainly from the external carotid artery via the distal branches of the internal maxillary artery. A smaller contribution comes from the anterior and posterior ethmoidal arteries which are branches of the ophthalmic artery, itself a branch of the internal carotid artery.
- Most cases can be managed conservatively with nasal packing or local cautery. Intractable epistaxis which fails to respond to conservative measures can be treated with transarterial embolisation of the internal maxillary artery using microparticles or platinum coils as an alternative to surgical ligation.

5.2.5 Obstetric Haemorrhage

- Embolisation has a major role to play in the management of obstetric haemorrhage which remains an important cause of maternal mortality worldwide.
- Embolisation is now established as a safe and highly effective treatment for postpartum haemorrhage and has the advantage of uterine preservation when compared to hysterectomy.
- Prophylactic temporary balloon occlusion of the internal iliac arteries is also performed in patients with placenta accreta to minimise haemorrhagic complications during delivery.

5.3 Patient Preparation

- Appropriate patient resuscitation and stabilisation with maintenance of airway, breathing and circulation.
- Multidisciplinary involvement of the anaesthetics, surgical, medical, trauma or obstetric teams in resuscitation and further management is essential in all cases.

- At least two large bore intravenous access for IV fluid infusion, sedation and resuscitation measures.
- Blood investigations including a contemporaneous full blood count, renal function tests and coagulation studies. For maximum benefit from embolisation, systemic coagulopathy should be corrected.

5.4 Case Examples

Case 5.1

A 45 year old female patient fell from a horse and sustained blunt trauma to her left flank. She was in hypovolaemic shock on arrival to the Emergency Department and was resuscitated with intravenous fluids. She underwent an urgent CT of the abdomen which revealed a large left perinephric haematoma and active arterial bleeding from the lower pole of the left kidney (Fig. 5.2). She was transferred to the interventional radiology suite for embolisation of this bleeding arterial branch. (Fig. 5.3).

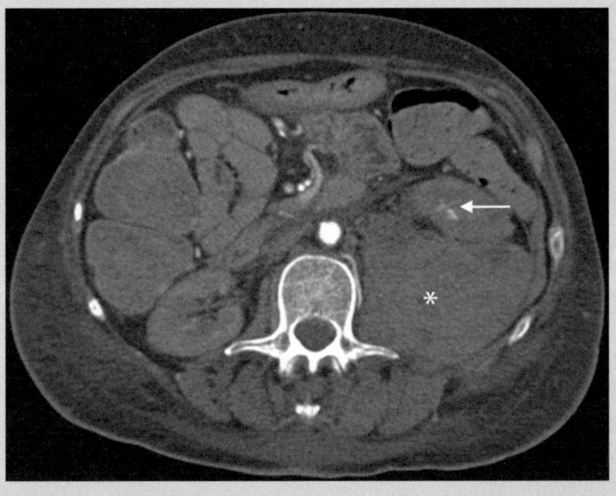

Fig. 5.2 Contrast enhanced arterial phase CT of the abdomen showing anterior displacement of the left kidney by a large perinephric haematoma (*asterisk*). There is a focus of active arterial haemorrhage in the lower pole of the left kidney (*arrow*)

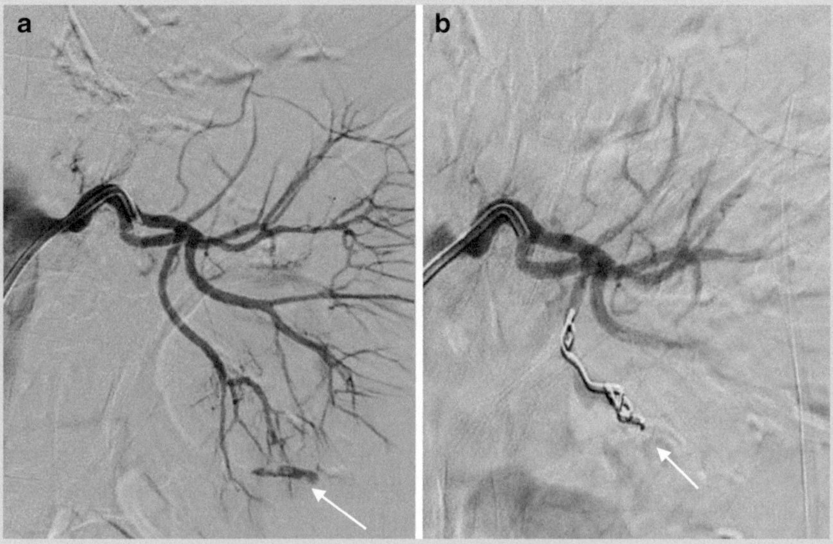

Fig. 5.3 (**a**) Following right common femoral arterial access, a 5 French catheter was used to selectively catheterise the left renal artery. Angiography showed active extravasation of contrast from a lower pole branch of the left renal artery (*arrow*). (**b**) This branch was selected with a catheter and embolised with metallic coils resulting in immediate cessation of haemorrhage (*arrow*). She made an uneventful recovery and avoided the need for invasive surgery or nephrectomy

Case 5.2

A 70 year old female patient fell down a flight of stairs at home and sustained multiple left sided rib fractures. She complained of severe left sided lower chest and upper abdominal pain and underwent an urgent CT of the abdomen at presentation to the Emergency Department which showed splenic lacerations associated with multiple pseudoaneurysms which were at high risk of rupture. She was transferred to the Interventional Radiology suite for further management (Figs. 5.4 and 5.5).

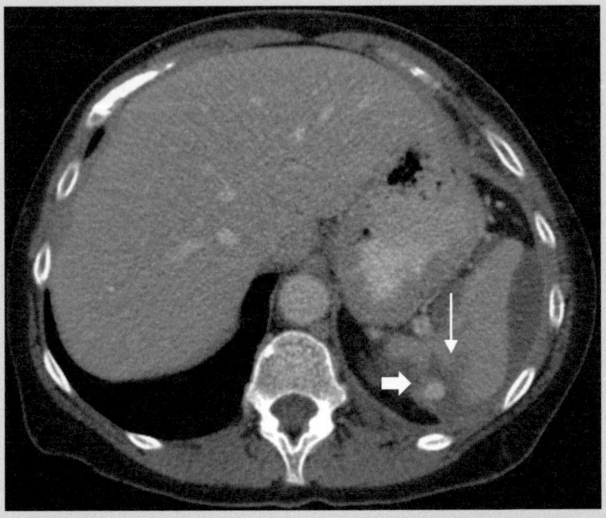

Fig. 5.4 Contrast enhanced CT of the upper abdomen showing a splenic laceration with contained perisplenic haematoma (*arrow*) and pseudoaneurysms arising from distal splenic arterial branches (*thick arrow*)

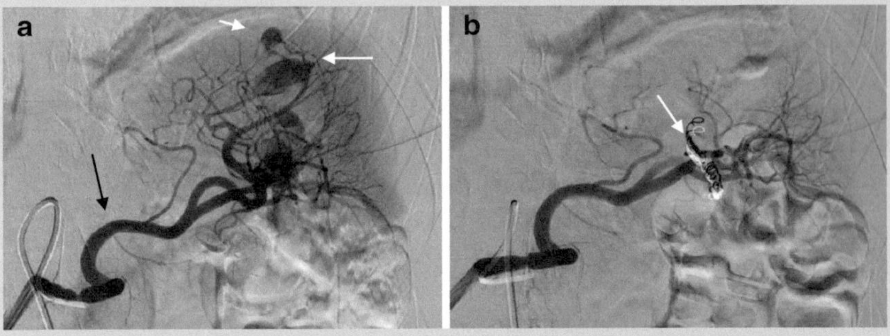

Fig. 5.5 (**a**) Following arterial access, the splenic artery (*black arrow*) was catheterised and angiography confirmed multiple traumatic pseudoaneurysms (*white arrows*), fed by distal branches of the splenic artery. (**b**) These branches were embolised with metallic coils to occlude the pseudoaneurysms (*arrow*). Although the superior pole of the spleen was sacrified in the process, a significant amount of normal splenic tissue was preserved and was sufficient to maintain splenic immune function. The patient recovered well from the procedure and was discharged home 2 days later

5.5 Complications

- Access site complications including haematoma, dissection, perforation (5–10%).
- Failure of embolisation – may be due to widespread coagulopathy such as disseminated intravascular coagulation from severe haemorrhage.

- Organ infarction.
- Non-target embolisation of other viscera.
- Mortality – variable depending on clinical status and extent of injury, in many cases these procedures are life-saving.

5.6 Results and Post-procedure Care

- In most cases, technical success is high and clinical success is apparent almost immediately after embolisation which may be reflected by haemodynamic stabilisation or discontinuation of bleeding on angiography.
- The aim of embolisation is to preserve as much of the injured organ as possible (such as in Cases 5.1 and 5.2) however occasionally it may be necessary to sacrifice the entire organ to preserve life. Some organs such as the spleen tolerate embolisation well and preserve sufficient splenic function due to perfusion from collateral vessels.
- Patients should be managed by a multidisciplinary team and depending on the overall clinical status, may require further care in an intensive care unit or additional surgical treatment for other injuries such as skeletal fractures.

Key Points

- Embolisation is an image-guided technique used to occlude vascular supply to organs using a variety of embolic materials.
- Acute embolisation procedures can be life-saving in a variety of situations including trauma, uncontrolled respiratory or gastrointestinal tract haemorrhage, intractable epistaxis and obstetric haemorrhage.
- Prompt imaging and early involvement of the Interventional Radiology service is key to identifying patients who may benefit from embolisation therapy, preserving life and visceral function.

Further Reading

1. Chakraverty S, Flood K, Kessel D, et al. CIRSE guidelines: quality improvement guidelines for endovascular treatment of traumatic hemorrhage. Cardiovasc Intervent Radiol. 2012;35:472–82.
2. Society of Interventional Radiology Standards of Practice Committee. Quality Improvement Guidelines for Percutaneous Transcatheter Embolization. Available at: http://www.sirweb.org/clinical/cpg/QI7.pdf.

6 Elective Embolisation Procedures

Hong Kuan Kok and Mark F. Given

6.1 Introduction

- Elective embolisation procedures encompass the minimally-invasive treatment of a diverse range of oncologic and non-oncologic conditions. This chapter will focus on the treatment of non-oncologic conditions including uterine fibroids, benign prostatic hyperplasia and gonadal vein embolisation (varicocoele and pelvic varicosities seen in pelvic congestion syndrome). Embolisation of tumours and vascular malformations will be covered in subsequent chapters.
- The embolic materials available to the Interventional Radiologist include specially designed devices such as metallic coils and vascular plugs, microparticles, gelatine sponges and liquid agents such as glue, thrombin or non-adhesive liquid embolics (ethylene vinyl alcohol copolymer).

6.2 Clinical Scenarios

6.2.1 Uterine Fibroid Embolisation

- Uterine fibroids or leiomyomas are very common benign smooth muscle tumours of the uterus. They may be asymptomatic or result in symptoms including menorrhagia, dysmenorrhoea and infertility. When sufficiently large, fibroids can also

H.K. Kok (✉)
Department of Radiology, Beaumont Hospital and Royal College of Surgeons in Ireland, Dublin, Ireland
e-mail: terrykok@gmail.com

M.F. Given
Department of Radiology, Beaumont Hospital, Dublin, Ireland

H.K. Kok et al. (eds.), *Interventional Radiology for Medical Students*,
DOI 10.1007/978-3-319-53853-2_6

compress on adjacent pelvic viscera such as the urinary bladder and rectum leading to pressure symptoms manifesting as urinary frequency or incomplete bladder and bowel emptying.

- Management of symptomatic fibroids include medical therapy with analgesics and hormones, surgery (myomectomy or hysterectomy) and increasingly, minimally-invasive uterine sparing procedures such as uterine fibroid embolisation (UFE).
- UFE is an established endovascular procedure with high success rates (>90%) for the treatment of symptomatic fibroids. It is now recommended as a first-line treatment option alongside surgical treatment in various guidelines including those from the National Institute for Health and Care Excellence (NICE) in the United Kingdom, conjoint recommendations from the Royal College of Obstetricians & Gynaecologists and the Royal College of Radiologists as well as the American College of Obstetricians & Gynecologists (ACOG).
- UFE is performed as a day or short stay (overnight) procedure and involves selective catheterisation of both uterine arteries and flow-directed embolisation with microparticles ranging in size from 500 to 900 microns.
- Many patients experience improvement in symptoms within 2–3 weeks following UFE and benefits are sustained in a large majority of patients. A small proportion (15–20%) may require re-intervention either with repeat UFE or surgery in the 5 year period following UFE.

6.2.2 Prostate Artery Embolisation

- Similar to UFE, prostate artery embolisation (PAE) has recently emerged as an alternative to surgical treatment in patients with benign prostatic hyperplasia. Symptoms of benign prostatic hyperplasia may include urinary frequency, urgency, poor stream, dribbling and urinary retention requiring catheterisation.
- Although experience is limited, early studies have shown that PAE can reduce prostate volumes between 20–40% with improvement in maximum urinary flow rates and reduction in post-void urinary retention.
- At present, PAE is performed in select centres with sufficient experience in this procedure, often in the context of clinical research. Further large-scale studies are awaited before PAE can be adopted as a mainstream procedure.

6.2.3 Gonadal Vein Embolisation

- Gonadal vein embolisation is performed for the treatment of symptomatic varicocoeles in men. Varicocoeles are dilated veins of the pampiniform venous plexus in the scrotum and occur more commonly on the left side. They may

result in pain and discomfort, particularly after long periods of standing. A small proportion of varicocoeles also result in subfertility.
- Embolisation of the testicular vein on the affected side with metallic coils, sclerosant material or glue is a highly effective treatment provided that the clinical symptoms are attributable to the varicocoele.
- Dilated pelvic varicosities in females, which are analogous to varicocoeles in men can result in pelvic congestion syndrome. Symptoms include chronic pelvic pain which is typically worse at the end of the day or after long periods of standing. Patients may also have co-existing vulval varices. Embolisation of the gonadal veins and dilated varicosities can be highly effective in improving symptoms in carefully selected patients.

6.2.4 Other Embolisation Procedures

- Virtually any organ system in the body can be treated by embolisation and there is a wide spectrum of procedures that can be performed.
- Examples include:
  - Endoleak embolisation following endovascular aneurysm repair (EVAR).
  - Embolisation of visceral artery aneurysms in the splanchnic circulation.
  - Tumour embolisation such as benign (angiomyolipoma) and malignant (renal cell carcinoma) renal tumours.
  - Portal vein embolisation prior to hepatic resection to promote hypertrophy of the future liver remnant after resection.
  - Embolisation of vascular (e.g. arteriovenous malformation) and lymphatic malformations.
  - Embolisation of gastric varices via balloon-occluded retrograde transvenous obliteration (BRTO) technique.
  - Bariatric embolisation – under investigation.

6.3 Patient Preparation

- Discussion at a multidisciplinary meeting or clinic review with comprehensive assessment of symptoms, signs, investigations and imaging with input from referring clinicians (e.g. Gynaecologists, Urologists) and Interventional Radiology.
- Can be performed as a day or short-stay procedure.
- Fasting for at least 6 hours prior to the procedure.
- Assess for any history of medication allergies which may preclude administration of iodinated contrast agents.
- Intravenous access, ideally at least 18 gauge for IV fluid infusion, conscious sedation and resuscitation measures if necessary.

- Blood investigations including a contemporaneous full blood count, renal function tests and coagulation studies. Most operators would use a cut-off international normalised ratio (INR) of less than 1.5 and platelet count of greater than 50,000.
- Prophylactic antibiotic cover with adequate analgesia for UFE as post-embolisation pain can be severe in the first 2–3 h following the procedure. This typically lasts between 8 to 12 h and many patients are admitted for overnight pain management and observation. Some centres use epidural analgesia, superior hypogastric nerve blocks or opioid based patient controlled analgesia pumps to minimise patient discomfort.

6.4 Case Examples

Case 6.1

A 42-year-old female patient with uterine fibroids was referred from her Gynaecologist with severe menorrhagia and irregular periods requiring intermittent blood transfusions for anaemia. She wished to avoid invasive surgery and also expressed a desire to maintain her uterus and chose to undergo UFE. (Figs. 6.1 and 6.2).

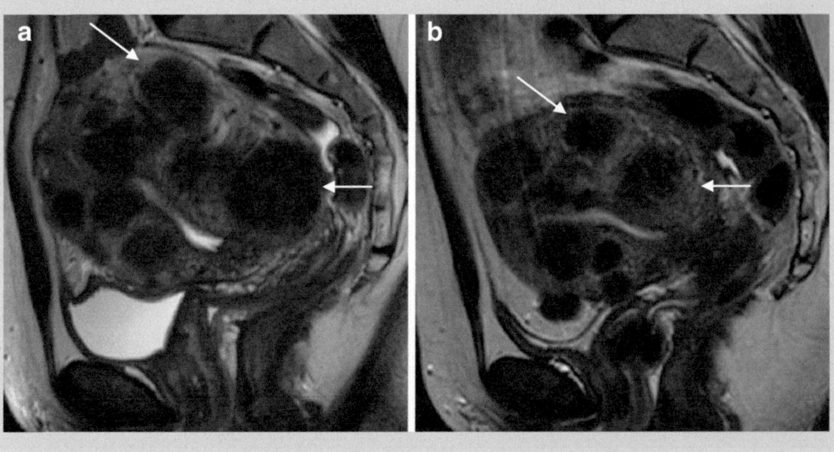

Fig. 6.1 (**a**) Pre-procedure MRI was performed showing an enlarged uterus containing multiple T2-hypointense fibroids (*arrows*). These were suitable for UFE and the patient returned for treatment 2 weeks after her MRI. (**b**) Follow-up MRI 6 months after embolisation showing decrease in size of multiple fibroids (*arrows*)

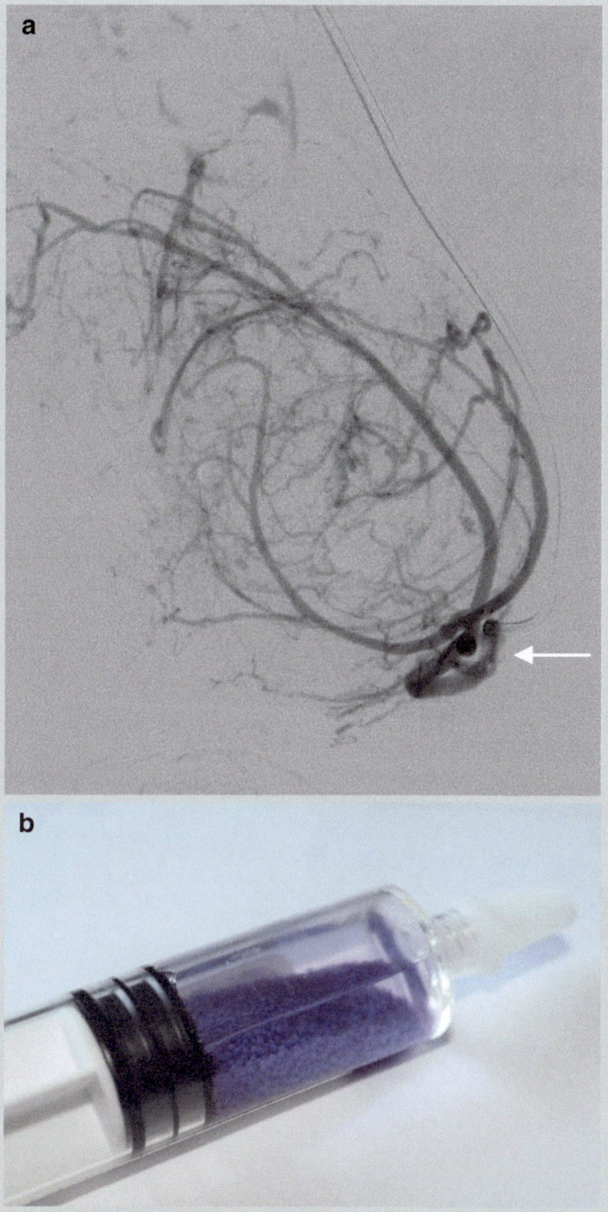

Fig. 6.2 (**a**) Following arterial access through the right common femoral artery, the left uterine artery (*arrow*) was selectively catheterised with a microcatheter and angiography confirmed avid vascular supply to the enlarged fibroid uterus. (**b**) Both uterine arteries were embolised with permanent calibrated microparticles (700 micron particles in this case). Her symptoms improved within a week of her procedure and a follow-up MRI at 6 months confirmed complete devascularisation of the fibroids with reduction in uterine size

Case 6.2

A 38 year old man was referred by his Urologist with dull aching pain in the left scrotum, worse at the end of the day. Clinical examination revealed a soft swelling separate from the left testicle and a scrotal ultrasound confirmed a moderate size varicocoele with augmentation of flow in the veins with the Valsalva manoeuvre (Fig. 6.3). As his symptoms were affecting his job, which involved prolonged periods of standing, he opted for varicocoele embolisation and was admitted to the IR day ward for the procedure. (Fig. 6.4).

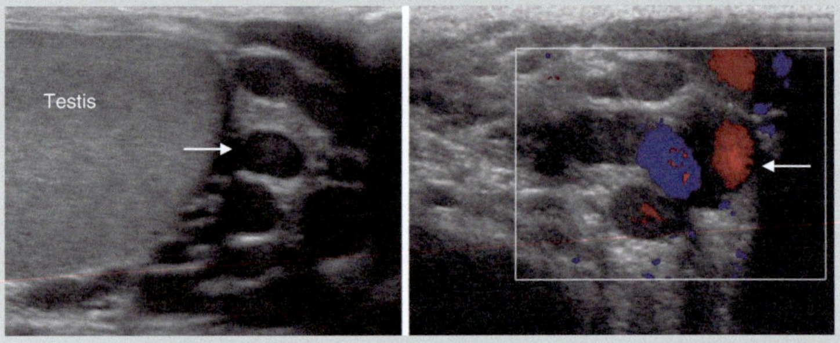

Fig. 6.3 Scrotal ultrasound showing enlarged veins with hypervascular flow on colour Doppler in the left scrotum consistent with varicocoele (*arrows*)

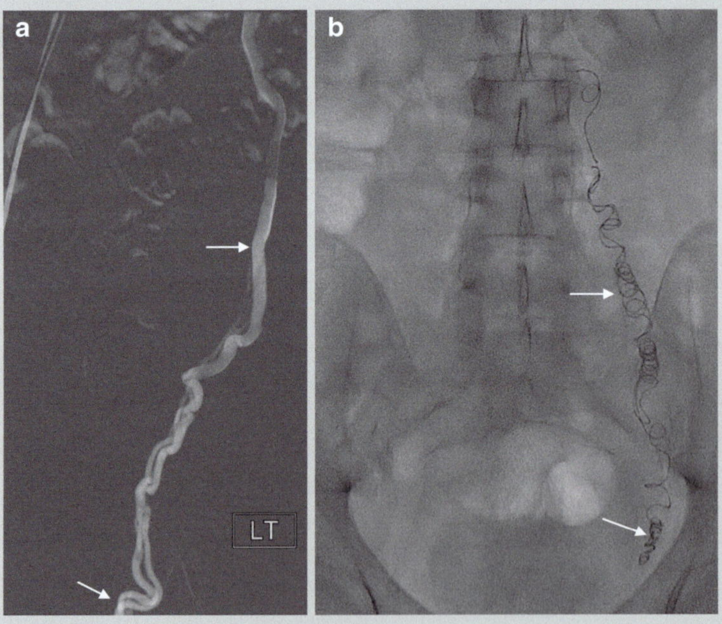

Fig. 6.4 (**a**) Following access via the right common femoral vein, a catheter was advanced up the IVC, into the left renal vein and subsequently, the left testicular vein (which drains into the left renal vein). Venography confirmed an enlarged left testicular vein and varicocoele (*arrows*). (**b**) Multiple metallic coils were placed throughout the length of the testicular vein (*arrows*) resulting in complete occlusion of the vein. His symptoms improved within the first week and completely resolved at 6 week follow-up

6.5 Complications

- Access site complications including haematoma, dissection, perforation.
- Pain – particularly following UFE which can be severe.
- Infection (2.5%).
- Failure or need for repeat embolisation due to recurrence of symptoms.
- Organ infarction (very rare).
- Non-target embolisation of other viscera.
- Post-embolisation syndrome (3%) which consists of a constellation of symptoms including fever, pain, nausea and vomiting, typically occurring within the first 48–72 h of embolisation. These symptoms may be confused with infection but this can be anticipated, particularly with embolisation of large fibroids or tumours.
- Amenorrhoea following UFE (4%).

6.6 Post-procedure Care and Review

- If performed via arterial access (e.g. UFE or PAE), bed rest for 4–6 h following the procedure with gradual mobilisation soon after. Bed rest and observation for 1–2 h following venous access is usually sufficient.
- Observation of vital signs and access site for local complications including haematoma and pseudoaneurysm formation.
- Commencement of appropriate analgesics following UFE for pain control.
- Clinical follow-up after embolisation to assess response. Follow-up imaging is also typically arranged for patients undergoing UFE with a repeat MRI at 6 months to assess for procedural success and uterine size.

Key Points

- Embolisation is an image-guided technique used to occlude vascular supply to organs with a variety of embolic materials.
- Elective embolisation procedures involve treatment of a variety of oncologic and non-oncologic conditions such as uterine fibroids, benign prostatic hyperplasia, varicoclele and pelvic congestion syndrome, sparing the need for more invasive surgical treatment.
- UFE and gonadal vein embolisation are highly effective (90%) and are accepted first-line treatment options for symptomatic fibroids or varicocoeles.
- PAE is an emerging and promising technique for treatment of benign prostatic hyperplasia.
- Adequate pain control and observation for post-embolisation syndrome is particularly important in patients undergoing UFE.

Further Reading

1. NICE interventional procedure guidance [IPG367]. Uterine artery embolisation for fibroids. Available at: https://www.nice.org.uk/guidance/ipg367.
2. Society of Interventional Radiology Standards of Practice Committee. Quality Improvement Guidelines for Percutaneous Transcatheter Embolization. Available at: http://www.sirweb.org/clinical/cpg/QI7.pdf.
3. van Overhagen H, Reekers JA. Uterine artery embolization for symptomatic Leiomyomata. Cardiovasc Intervent Radiol. 2015;38:536–42.

Vascular Malformations and Treatment

7

Elizabeth Ryan and Mark F. Given

7.1 Introduction

- These are endothelial malformations which may be arterial, venous, capillary, lymphatic or mixed (e.g. arteriovenous).
- They are uncommonly encountered and treatment is complex. Patients with vascular malformations are best managed in an expert centre via a multidisciplinary approach by experienced clinicians incorporating input from different specialties including IR, Dermatology and Plastic surgery.
- They are divided into low and high-flow lesions. Low-flow lesions include venous, capillary, lymphatic or mixed malformations without arterial supply. High-flow malformations involve an arterial component.
- Pre-treatment characterisation with diagnostic imaging is mandatory as low and high-flow lesions are managed differently. MRI and ultrasound are the most commonly employed diagnostic modalities.

Imaging is also important for delineating the anatomy of the lesion and its proximity to or involvement of adjacent structures.

E. Ryan (✉)
Department of Radiology, Beaumont Hospital and Royal College of Surgeons in Ireland, Dublin, Ireland
e-mail: lizryan1@gmail.com

M.F. Given
Department of Radiology, Beaumont Hospital, Dublin, Ireland

H.K. Kok et al. (eds.), *Interventional Radiology for Medical Students*,
DOI 10.1007/978-3-319-53853-2_7

7.2 Low-Flow Lesions

- Venous, capillary, lymphatic and mixed malformations consist of multiple venous channels in a hamartomatous stroma connecting to and draining via normal veins.
- Many malformations present with swelling, pain and/or haemorrhage. Restricted movement, deformity or aesthetic appearance may also prompt presentation, depending on the size, extent and location of the malformation.
- **Percutaneous sclerotherapy** is the treatment for choice for most low-flow malformations and is usually performed with a liquid sclerosant such as sodium tetradecyl sulphate (STD) or ethanol.

7.2.1 Indications

- Pain, swelling, haemorrhage or aesthetic considerations
- Platelet consumption

7.2.2 Alternative Treatment Options

Conservative	Patients may not consider the lesion particularly troublesome and may be satisfied with reassurance that it is benign and not life-threatening. If so, conservative management is a reasonable option. However, it is important to inform the patient (and parents in young children) that, in contrast to haemangiomas, vascular malformations will not regress with age and may enlarge.
Surgical resection	For small superficial lesions. Often recur.
Laser	For capillary vascular malformations.
Radiotherapy	Rarely used due to limited efficacy and skin changes.

7.2.3 Contraindications

- Known right-to-left shunts, e.g. patent foramen ovale. These risk embolisation of the sclerosant into the arterial circulation which could be catastrophic.

7.2.4 Patient Preparation

- **Imaging** Should be reviewed prior to the procedure to confirm it is a low-flow malformation, select an access route and identify involved or adjacent structures.
- **Lab** Full blood count, coagulation status. International normalised ratio should be <1.5 and platelets $>50 \times 10^9$/L.

- **Medications** Clopidogrel/warfarin/novel anticoagulant medications should be held for a duration appropriate to the specific agent.
- **Fasting** Clear fluids are allowed up to 2 h prior to the procedure; fasting for all other intake for at least 4 h.
- **IV access**
- **Anaesthesia** These procedures are painful and adequate analgesia and sedation are required. General anaesthesia is often used.
- **Written informed consent** should be documented after discussed of the procedure and its benefits, risks and alternatives.

7.2.5 Technique

- Patient positioning is appropriate to the location of lesion and the access route. Sterile field.
- Some operators advocate catheter angiography at the time of first intervention in order to confirm its low-flow status prior to percutaneous treatment and also provides a baseline angiographic study for future comparison.
- Placement of a 21G needle into the malformation under ultrasound guidance.
- Injection of contrast under digital subtraction angiography, noting the volume and rate of contrast material required to reach a draining vein.
- Sclerosant is then mixed with contrast medium and carefully injected at the desired volume and rate under imaging guidance.
- Treatment may require several sessions depending on the lesion size. On each session up to three small areas of the lesion are treated in order to keep the post-procedure swelling to an acceptable level and reduce the risk of skin ulceration.

7.2.6 Post-procedural Care

Analgesia as required.

Swelling is expected and may take several weeks to resolve. It is important to counsel the patient prior to treatment that swelling may transiently increase after treatment. Furthermore, the lesion may take up to several months to fibrose and shrink in response to sclerosant administration. Occasionally, a short course of corticosteroids can be prescribed to reduce post-treatment swelling.

7.2.7 Complications

- Skin ulceration (8%)
- Neurovascular damage (2–5%)
- Muscle atrophy or contracture (<1%)
- Dissemination via draining veins resulting in arrhythmias, DVT, pulmonary emboli, compartment syndrome (rare)

7.3 High-Flow Lesions

- Any malformation with an arterial component, including arteriovenous malformations and arteriovenous fistulae.
- These represent a connection between the arterial and venous systems without an intervening capillary bed, resulting in high-flow through the channels.
- They present with local symptoms similar to low-flow malformations such as pain, swelling and sometimes haemorrhage.
- Additionally, they may produce systemic symptoms secondary to arteriovenous shunting including paradoxical emboli, high-output cardiac failure and ischaemia of the tissues peripheral to the shunt (e.g. in the extremities) as a result of flow diversion. These are more commonly associated with AV fistulae than AVMs, the latter having a complex nidus of small channels between arterial supply and venous drainage rather than a direct connection.
- These are treated with transarterial embolisation.

7.3.1 Indications

- Pain, swelling, aesthetic appearance.
- Shunting resulting in high-output cardiac failure or peripheral ischaemia.
- Platelet consumption.

7.3.2 Alternative Therapies

- **Conservative**
- **Surgical** resection of small superficial malformations is feasible but they commonly recur.

7.3.3 Contraindications

- Right-to-left shunt, for example a patent foramen ovale. (relative contraindication)

7.3.4 Patient Preparation

- **Imaging** Should be reviewed prior to the procedure to confirm the diagnosis, identify the supplying arteries and other structures either involved by the lesion or sharing the same arterial supply (risk of non-target embolisation).
- **Lab** Full blood count, coagulation status. International normalised ratio should be <1.5 and platelets $>50 \times 10^9$/L.

- **Medications** Clopidogrel/warfarin/novel anticoagulant medications should be held for a duration appropriate to the specific agent.
- **Fasting** Clear fluids are allowed up to 2 h prior to the procedure; fasting for all other intake for at least 4 h.
- **IV access**
- **Anaesthesia** These procedures may be painful and adequate analgesia and sedation are required. General anaesthesia may be necessary, especially in younger patients.
- **Written informed consent** should be documented after discussed of the procedure and its benefits, risks and alternatives.

7.3.5 Technique

- Supine position, sterile field.
- Right common femoral artery needle access, placement of a guidewire and sheath.
- The supplying artery is accessed with a standard catheter and wire, and selective access into the small arterial branches is performed with a microcatheter.
- It is critical to deliver the embolic agent into the centre (or "nidus") of the malformation. Embolisation of larger, more proximal branches without embolising the nidus results in recruitment of new arterial supply and treatment failure.
- Liquid embolic agents such as glue, ethanol or Onyx (ethylene vinyl alcohol copolymer) are used. A combination of agents may be used to treat the nidus and feeding arteries.
- Sometimes balloon occlusion of the venous outflow (via a separate venous access) is performed to reduce the flow and prevent rapid "wash out" or dissemination of the embolic agent.

7.3.6 Post-procedural Care

- As for all arterial access, bed rest for 6 h and regular observation for bleeding at the puncture site.
- Analgesia as required.

7.3.7 Complications

- Complications related to arterial puncture including haemorrhage and pseudoaneurysm formation. (1–5%).
- Non-target embolisation, the sequelae of which are specific to the treatment site. (complication rate also specific to treatment site).

Case

This 4-year-old boy presented with an enlarging, visible and intermittently painful vascular malformation involving his left upper limb. Workup confirmed a low-flow lesion safe for percutaneous sclerotherapy.

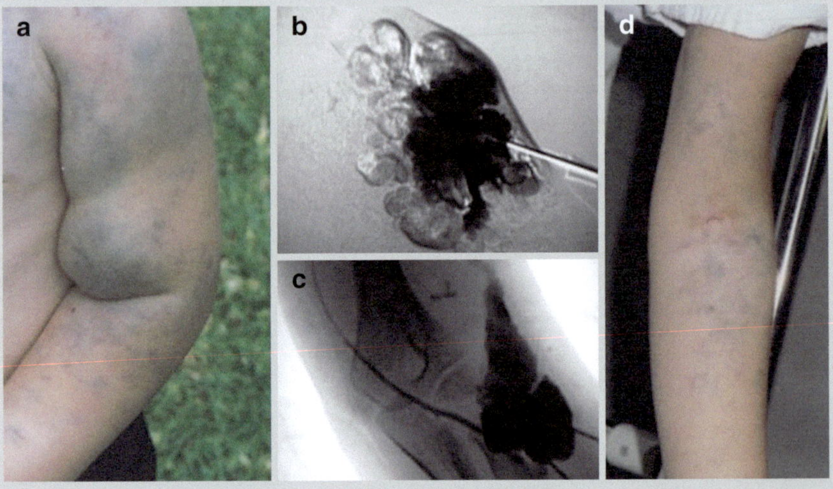

Percutaneous sclerotherapy of upper limb vascular malformation. (**a**) Multiple visible and palpable distended veins in the left arm. (**b**) and (**c**) Direct puncture and contrast injection under fluoroscopy allows visualisation of the malformation and injection of sclerosant. (**d**) One year and several sclerotherapy treatments later, the malformation has significantly decreased in size and is less visible. The patient's symptoms had also improved

Key Points

- Vascular malformations are uncommon and treatment may be complex and include staged or multi-modal therapy. They should be evaluated and managed in a specialist centre by experienced operators.
- They should be correctly characterised as low-flow or high-flow lesions prior to treatment in order to select the appropriate treatment method.
- Pre-procedure imaging is typically via ultrasound and/or MRI.
- Treatment carries risk and conservative management is a valid option if the malformation is not particularly troublesome.

Suggested Reading

1. Markovic JN, Shortell CE. Multidisciplinary treatment of extremity arteriovenous malformations. J Vasc Surg Venous Lymphat Disord. 2015;3(2):209–18.
2. Transcatheter Embolisation and Therapy. Kessel and Ray (Editors). Lee and Watkinson (Series Editors). (Springer 2010).

Venous Access Principles and Devices (PICC, Vascular Access Ports and Tunneled Catheters)

8

Timothy Murray, Hong Kuan Kok, and Michael Lee

8.1 Introduction

- Venous access is a mainstay of hospital-based patient treatment, and is increasingly used in community-based treatment. Peripheral venous cannulae have a short lifespan. In addition, the limited gauge of smaller peripheral veins reduces permissible flow rates. As such, these small, low-flow vessels are more prone to venous sclerosis from certain intravenous medications and other substances compared to larger, high-flow veins.
- Central venous access is indicated in patients who require intermediate-long term access for treatment such as antibiotics, chemotherapy and haemodialysis.
- The choice of access site and type of vascular access device depends on the clinical indication, expected duration of treatment and patient status. A variety of device types are available which vary in terms of size, lumen number, catheter length, material, coating and termination (hub, port reservoir, etc.). These are tailored to the patient and the clinical indication. Additionally, some catheter designs feature both anti-microbial and heparin-impregnated materials which have additional benefits.
- Common venous access sites for catheter insertion include the internal jugular and femoral veins. The basilic, cephalic and brachial veins in the arm are also commonly used for placement of peripherally-inserted central catheters (PICC).

T. Murray
Department of Radiology, Beaumont Hospital, Dublin, Ireland
e-mail: murraytim0@gmail.com

H.K. Kok • M. Lee (✉)
Department of Radiology, Beaumont Hospital and Royal College of Surgeons in Ireland, Dublin, Ireland

H.K. Kok et al. (eds.), *Interventional Radiology for Medical Students*,
DOI 10.1007/978-3-319-53853-2_8

8.2 Procedure Indications

- Requirement for prolonged intravenous medications, such as antimicrobials in prosthetic joint infections, osteomyelitis, endocarditis and ventriculitis.
- Administration of substances not suitable to the peripheral venous route due to risk of sclerosis or extravasation, such as total parenteral nutrition, chemotherapy and hyper/hypoosmolar solutions.
- Monitoring of central venous pressures.
- Lack of suitable peripheral access (often in long-stay patients following serial phlebotomy and cannulation, or in patients with subcutaneous oedema or obesity).
- PICC lines are appropriate for short-to-intermediate durations (days to weeks). Patients requiring over 30 days access may benefit from a tunneled catheter due to lower infection risk.
- Prolonged regular outpatient therapy, such as chemotherapy or antibiotics may benefit from implanted vascular access ports (also known as Portacaths). These devices have lower infection rates and have less restriction on activities of daily living, such as showering or swimming.
- Wide-bore access such as tunneled catheters are used when high-flow venous access is required in haemodialysis and plasmapheresis. As regular, prolonged venous access is required, these lines are tunneled under the skin, with only the catheter hubs visible externally for access.

8.3 Procedure Contraindications

- No suitable vein for access due to thrombosis or occlusion
- Infection or cellulitis in the overlying cutaneous access site
- Uncontrolled systemic sepsis (relative)
- Systemic coagulopathy (relative)

8.4 Patient Preparation

- Review indication, required duration and patient-specific factors to ensure appropriate device selection. Patient counselling regarding the immediate and long-term care of the access device.
- Assess for allergies including intolerance to adhesives and dressings (certain devices such as PICC lines require prolonged use of adhesives and skin dressings).
- PICC and non-tunneled central venous lines are inserted under local anaesthesia. Conscious sedation is reserved for tunneled access or port implantation, or in selected patients who may not tolerate the procedure due to anxiety or confusion.
- Where sedation is required, the patient should fast for at least 6 h and have appropriate peripheral intravenous access.
- Full blood count and coagulation screen should be performed in patients on anti-coagulation, with an underlying coagulopathy or when a tunneled device or port is being implanted. A target INR <1.5 and platelets count of $>50,000$ is generally

chosen by most operators. Coagulopathy is not an absolute contraindication as superficial access sites (e.g. for PICC) are easily compressible.
- The use of prophylactic pre-procedural antibiotics is not supported by current evidence.

8.5 Complications

- Overall risk of a major complication is <3%.
- Prolonged duration, heavy bacterial colonisation of the insertion site and catheter hub, and the use of groin access (femoral vein) are all associated with higher rates of complications.

Specific complications and incidences include:

- Infection, both cellulitis and central-line associated blood stream infection (CLASBI) (1–3% at time of procedure, incidence increases with duration)
- Venous thrombosis, stenosis or occlusion (4%)
- Arterial puncture (1–4%)
- Air embolus (1%)
- Pneumothorax / Haemothorax (1% incidence in subclavian / jugular puncture only)
- Haematoma (1–3%)
- Sedation-related cardiovascular complications and anaphylaxis.

8.6 Procedures

8.6.1 Non-tunneled Catheters (Including Central Lines and PICC)

- Following review of the clinical indication and duration, the appropriate vascular access device and insertion site are chosen. Written informed consent is obtained and the procedure is performed under strict sterile technique and imaging guidance.
- The patient is typically positioned supine on the fluoroscopy table. Using ultrasound guidance, the proposed puncture site is examined. The patency and calibre of the target vessel is assessed. Doppler imaging is used to assess the venous waveform and flow. Vessel compressibility, the presence of valves and examination of the vessel wall confirms both vessel patency and venous access rather than arterial access. Adjacent structures such as arteries, lymph nodes and organs are noted to avoid inadvertent puncture.
- Local anaesthesia is infiltrated at the access site. Using real-time ultrasound guidance and the Seldinger technique (See Chap. 3), a vascular access needle is advanced and the vein is punctured. Venous flashback is confirmed in the vessel hub by aspiration. A guidewire is then advanced through the needle into the vein. Fluoroscopy is used to track the position of the guidewire within the vein. Advancing the guidewire

tip across the diaphragm confirms appropriate placement within the venous system, along the path of the superior vena cava – right atrium – inferior vena cava and avoids inadvertent insertion into the azygos or collateral veins.

- The catheter length is chosen to allow placement of the tip at the cavoatrial junction. Larger devices typically require the use of fascial dilators to enlarge the venotomy tract to an appropriate width. The catheter is advanced, and the tip is positioned is confirmed with fluoroscopy.
- The catheter is aspirated and flushed to confirm appropriate function and the line is flushed and primed with heparinised sterile saline. The external portion of the line is sutured or secured in place using a skin-adhesive dressing.

8.6.2 Tunneled Catheters (Haemodialysis and Hickman Catheters)

- High-flow vascular access is required for procedures such as haemodialysis or plasmapheresis and requires larger diameter catheters, generally between 12 and 16 French size. These catheters are too large for a peripheral vein, and require a large central vein for insertion. The most common initial location is the right IJV, which has a wide diameter with a straight course leading to the right atrium.
- Once the jugular vein has been successfully punctured, a separate incision is made on the upper anterior chest wall. A tract through the subcutaneous soft tissue is created by blunt dissection and the catheter tip is passed along the subcutaneous chest wall tract to the venotomy site. The catheter tip is subsequently advanced through a peel-away sheath into the IJV and advanced to the level of the right atrium under fluoroscopic guidance.
- The catheter hub is then secured in place to the chest wall with anchoring sutures and the skin incision overlying the venous puncture site is sutured over. This tunneling improves device stability and reduces risk of infection.

8.6.3 Implanted Vascular Access Port (Portacath)

- Implantable ports are inserted using a similar technique as described above for tunneled line insertion. With a tunneled line, the catheter hub remains external to the patient. Implantable ports are completely buried within the chest wall soft tissue.
- A small incision is used to create a subcutaneous pocket which will accommodate the port reservoir (Fig. 8.1 arrowhead). Once the device is inserted, with the diaphragm of the port facing upwards for puncture, the overlying skin is sutured over. The port is then punctured through the skin using a Huber needle as required.
- As the port device is completely internalised in the body, there is a lower risk of infection and less impact on activities of daily living such as showering or swimming, compared to other catheters with exposed hubs which have to be kept dry.

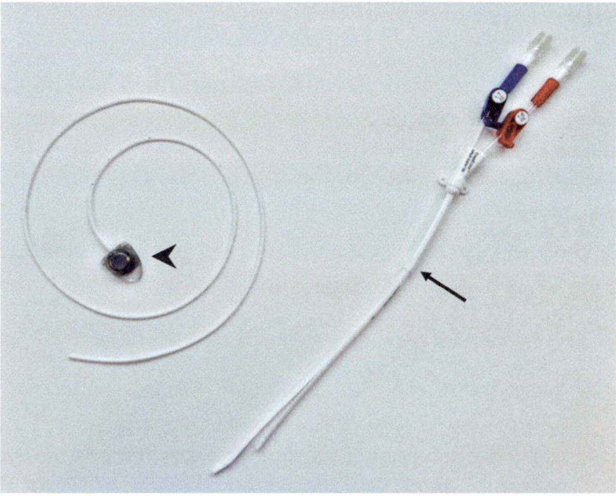

Fig. 8.1 Vascular access port (*left*) and tunneled dual-lumen haemodialysis catheter (*right*). Note the access port consists of a small diameter line (8 French) attached to a low-profile reservoir (*arrowhead*), allowing complete subcutaneous burial. The tunneled dialysis catheter is of larger diameter (14 French) has two lumens. The polyester cuff (*arrow*) anchors the line by causing formation of scar tissue and also provides a barrier against infection

8.7 Post Procedure Care and Review

- Haemostasis, line function and position should be checked at the end of each procedure by the operator. For tunneled or implantable port insertion, patients should be observed for 6 h in a recovery area or day ward if performed on an outpatient basis.
- The line should be primed and locked with an appropriate solution to prevent thrombosis after each use. Generally, heparinised saline is used for PICC lines and heparin or sodium citrate solutions for larger diameter lines depending on manufacturer's recommendations.
- Thrombolytic agents such as alteplase or urokinase may be helpful to restore potency to a nonfunctioning line.
- In patients with sepsis of unknown origin and an indwelling central venous line, negative blood cultures withdrawn from the line demonstrates a high negative predictive value of up to 98% in the exclusion of line sepsis. A "watchful wait" approach may be appropriate in this setting. Culture positive lines should be removed and sent for culture and sensitivity.
- PICC lines may be removed by non-specialist medical staff under sterile technique followed by compression to the access site to secure haemostasis.
- Removal of tunneled or implanted devices should only be performed by experienced personnel.

8.8 Results

- Success rates for image-guided placement of non-tunneled and tunneled central lines, PICC and implantable ports are all ≥95%.
- Rates of major morbidity at insertion are <3%.
- Rates of central line associated blood-stream infection (CLASBI) are 8.6 per 1000 catheter days.
- Rates of line thrombosis/occlusion are 1.2–3 per per 1000 catheter days.

Case

A 60-year old patient with end stage kidney disease secondary to diabetic nephropathy required vascular access for commencement of haemodialysis. He underwent insertion of a tunneled haemodialysis catheter in the Interventional Radiology angiographic suite (Fig. 8.2).

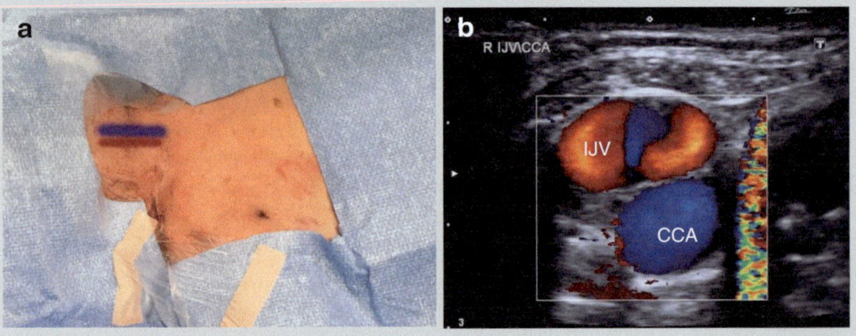

Fig. 8.2 Tunneled haemodialysis catheter insertion. (**a**) Patient positioned supine with the head turned to the left. A sterile drape has been placed over the right lower neck and upper chest. The approximate positions of the right internal jugular vein (IJV, *blue*) and common carotid artery (CCA, *red*) are indicated. (**b**) Duplex ultrasound of the neck vessels showing the IJV and CCA. (**c**) Under ultrasound guidance, the IJV is accessed with a 21 gauge micropuncture access needle (*arrow*). (**d**) Following access into the vein, a guidewire (*arrow*) is advanced into the IJV, superior vena cava and then into the inferior vena cava. Over the guidewire, serial fascial dilators are advanced through the venotomy site and a peel-away sheath is placed (*arrowhead*). (**e**) The tunneled dialysis catheter is passed subcutaneously through a "tunnel" formed by blunt dissection until its tip emerges at the level of the venotomy. (**f**) The catheter tip is then passed through the sheath until the entire catheter, except the access hubs, is internalised. The venotomy site is closed with a suture and the catheter is anchored to the skin with sutures. (**g**) Final position of the catheter tip within the right atrium (*arrow*) is confirmed on fluoroscopy

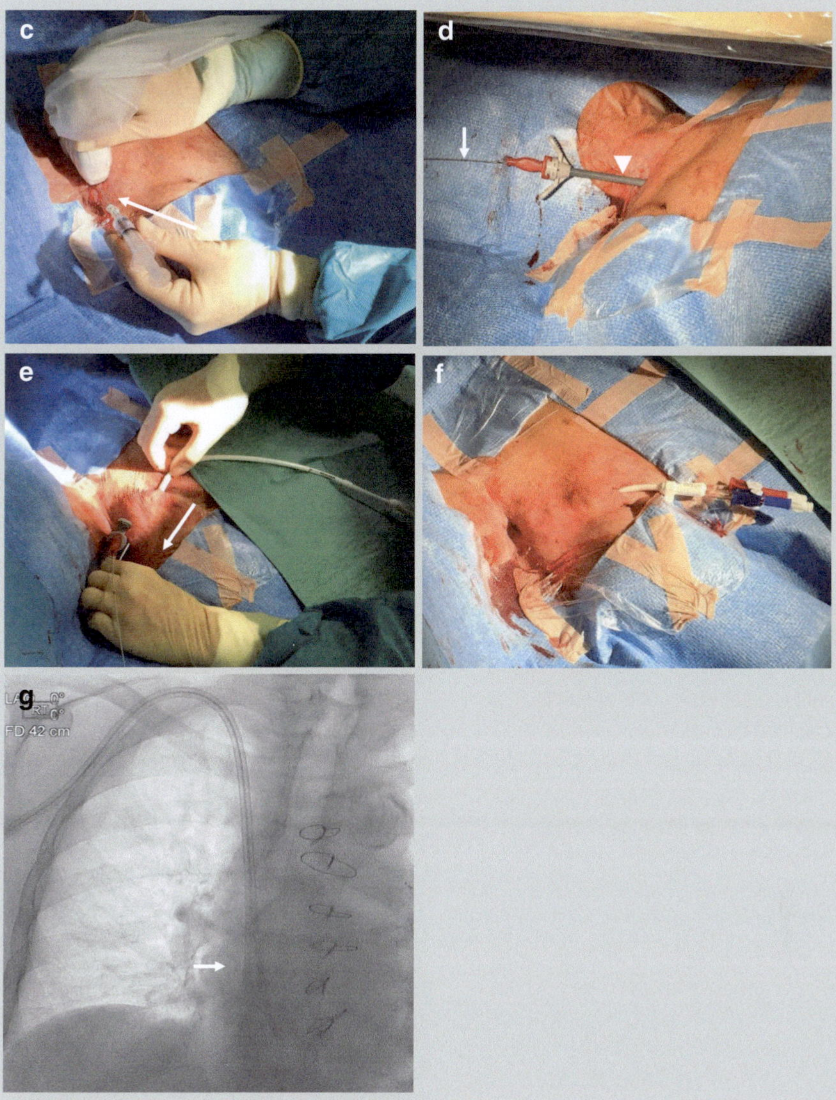

Fig. 8.2 (continued)

Key Points

- Venous access device placement either through a peripheral or central vein can be safely performed for a variety of clinical indications.
- The choice of venous access device and the site of insertion vary depending on clinical indication, duration of thera and individual patient factors.
- The use of imaging guidance such as ultrasound and fluoroscopy increases the safety of the procedure and minimises the risk of inadvertent arterial puncture, injury of surrounding structures and device malpositioning.
- Overall complication rates are low. The most commonly encountered intermediate to long-term complications include infection and thrombosis, both of which relate to the site and duration of device insertion.

Further Reading

1. Graham AS, Ozment C, Tegtmeyer K, Lai S, Braner DAV. Central venous catheterization. N Engl J Med. 2007;356(21):e21.
2. Marschall J, Mermel LA, Fakih M, et al. Strategies to prevent central line-associated bloodstream infections in acute care hospitals: 2014 update. Infect Control Hosp Epidemiol. 2014;35(7):753–71.

9 Venous Thromboembolism and IVC Filters

Michael Lee

9.1 Introduction

- 1.6 million people in the EU develop venous thromboembolism every year with 0.5 million deaths.
- More patients die in the UK from venous thromboembolism (VTE) than combined totals from breast cancer, road traffic accidents and AIDS (NICE 2009).
- VTE cost for Australia in 2008 was 3.9 Billion Dollars, which was more than the entire cancer treatment spend.
- Rudolf Virchow (1821–1902) bestowed the name embolus on venous thromboembolism in 1856 when he said "the detachment of larger or smaller fragments from the end of the softening thrombus, which are carried along be the current of blood and driven into remote vessels. This gives rise to the very frequent process on which I have bestowed the name (EMBOLIA)".
- Virchow also gave his name to Virchow's Triad, which predisposes to VTE, namely, hypercoagulable states, haemodynamic changes (stasis) and endothelial injury or dysfunction.
- Pulmonary emboli usually arise from thrombi that originate in the deep venous system of the lower extremities. They can also arise from pelvic, renal, upper extremity veins or right heart chambers.
- Treatment is by full anticoagulation for all patients suspected of having VTE. This is usually achieved by starting the patient on low molecular weighted Heparin (LMWH) with oral anticoagulation (Warfarin) initiated at the time of diagnosis and LMWH discontinued when the INR is 2.0 for at least 24 h, but no sooner than 5 days after Warfarin therapy has been commenced.

M. Lee
Department of Radiology, Beaumont Hospital and Royal College of Surgeons in Ireland, Dublin, Ireland
e-mail: mlee@rcsi.ie

H.K. Kok et al. (eds.), *Interventional Radiology for Medical Students*,
DOI 10.1007/978-3-319-53853-2_9

- In some patients, anticoagulation is either contraindicated or there has been a complication associated with anticoagulation so that it has to be stopped. An inferior vena cava (IVC) filter can be placed in these patients to protect against further pulmonary emboli.

9.2 Indications for IVC Filter

1. Patients with acute VTE with an absolute contraindication to anticoagulant therapy (e.g. recent surgery, haemorrhagic stroke, significant active or recent bleeding).
2. Patients who have documented recurrent VTE despite adequate anticoagulant therapy.
3. Originally, IVC filters were all permanent devices. In the last 15–20 years, retrievable devices have entered the market. These devices can be inserted percutaneously and removed once anticoagulation can be resumed. The retrievable filters have dramatically increased the rate of placement of IVC filters for prophylactic indications (trauma patients, bariatric surgery patients, patients pending surgery with a remote history of DVT or PE etc.). However, there is no evidence for placing IVC filters for VTE prophylaxis.

9.3 Contraindications

1. No femoral or jugular vein access – very rare
2. Septicemia

9.4 Patient Preparation

- Patients should be fasting from midnight of the previous day.
- A careful review of the indication should be performed to determine if the filter is warranted.
- Anticoagulation does not have to be stopped as the puncture site is venous.
- A decision should be made whether the filter is to be retrieved or would be or left as a permanent filter.
- If the filter is to be retrieved, a date should be set to retrieve the filter.
- Retrievable filters are best retrieved within 3 months of placement.

9.5 Procedure Description

1. IVC filters can be placed via the jugular veins or femoral veins. Some filters can be placed from an arm vein.

2. Ultrasound is used to puncture the femoral or jugular vein and a large sheath is placed into the inferior vena cava. Contrast material is injected through this sheath to measure the size of the cava and locate the level of the renal veins.
3. The IVC filter is released into the cava just below the level of the renal veins and is usually held in the caval wall by hooks, which are attached to the legs or arms of the filter.
4. A further injection of contrast material is performed to check centering in the cava and to ensure no thrombus has formed.
5. If the filter is to be retrieved, it is usually retrieved from the right jugular vein using a snare or a grasping forceps type device to snag the top of the filter. The filter is then retrieved by sliding a large sheath over the filter and removing it.

9.6 Filter Descriptions

- Many different filter designs are available. Most have hooks on some part of the filter structure that embed in the caval wall. This prevents migration.
- Most have an umbrella or conical type configuration.
- The filter comes with a large sheath through which the filter is placed and released in the cava.

9.7 Complications

1. Access site complications – haematoma and thrombosis <1%
2. Technical problems during insertion of insertion failure – 1–3%
3. IVC penetration by filter struts – 19%, usually asymptomatic
4. Filter migration to the heart-rare <1%
5. Filter fracture reported with certain types only <2%
6. IVC thrombosis with permanent filters – 4–8%

9.8 Filter Retrieval

- Retrieval rate is 92–95%
- If filters are placed with an intent to retrieve, the onus is on the IR service and referring clinical team to ensure that the filter is removed.
- Filters are generally removed via the right internal jugular vein using a snare or grasping forceps to engage the hook on the top of the filter.
- Filter tilt and endothelialisation (filter legs get incorporated into the caval wall) of the filter present difficulties for retrieval. Advanced techniques are available to remove these filters.
- The sooner the filter is retrieved, the better. Ideally filters should be removed within 3 months as the chances of success are highest in this time period (Fig. 9.1).

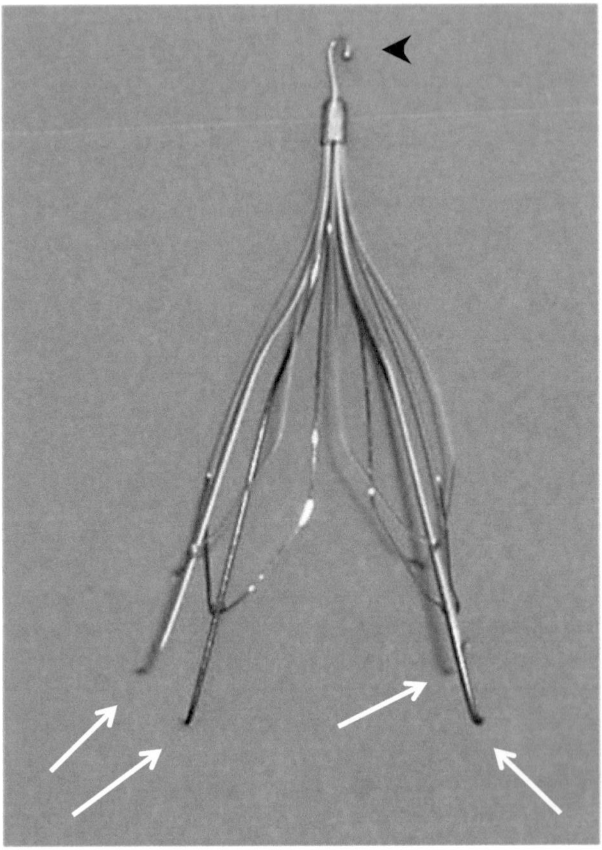

Fig. 9.1 Typical Conical Filter type. Note the hook on the top of the filter (*arrowhead*) for snaring and removal. Small hooks (*arrows*) are also seen on each of the legs that attach to filter to the caval wall

Case

A 30-year-old man with testicular cancer was referred for a retroperitoneal lymph node dissection for residual tumor post-chemotherapy. The surgery was uneventful but he developed a PE 3 days after surgery. Because of the recent surgery, he could not be anticoagulated and an IVC filter was placed. Six weeks later, when the patient was fully anticoagulated, the IVC filter was retrieved (Fig. 9.2).

Fig. 9.2 (**a**) Filter inerted in the IVC from the jugular route. (**b**) Six weeks later, the IVC filter was retrieved using a right jugular vein approach. A snare has been advanced through a long sheath and on this image, the hook on the end of the filter has been snared (*arrow*). (**c**) The sheath (*arrow*) is then advanced over the filter. (**d**) The sheath is then pushed down over the filter to collapse the filter and in this image the filter is now fully within the sheath and ready to be withdrawn. A final injection of contrast material is done to confirm that the cava has not been damaged and then the sheath is removed

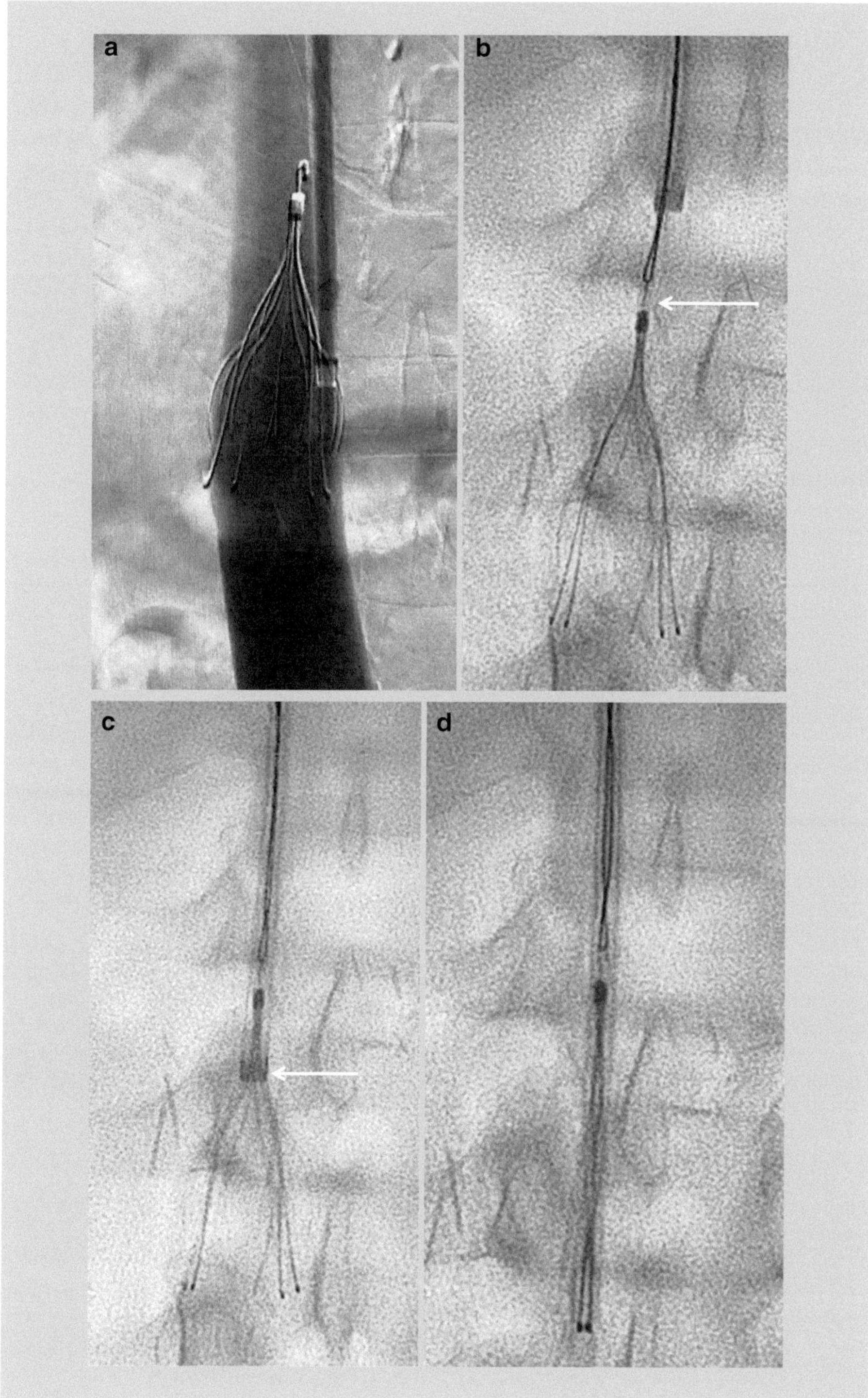
a
b
c
d

Key Points

- Venous thromboembolism (VTE) remains a significant healthcare problem throughout the World.
- IVC filters can be placed in patients with VTE who cannot receive anticoagulation or who have failed anticoagulation.
- Retrievable IVC filters can be placed in patients where there is a high risk of VTE where prophylaxis is required (before surgery if there is a remote history of VTE, multiple trauma patients, before bariatric surgery) and removed at a later date. However, evidence for prophylactic placement is limited.
- There is a 92%–95% success rate for removal if removed within 3 months of placement.

Suggested Reading

1. Brandjes DP, Buller HR, Heijboer H, et al. Randomised trial of effect of compression stockings in patients with symptomatic proximal-vein thrombosis. Lancet. 1997;349(9054):759–62.
2. Decousus H, Leizorovicz A, Parent F, et al. A clinical trial of vena caval filters in the prevention of pulmonary embolism in patients with proximal deep-vein thrombosis. N Engl J Med. 1998;338(7):409–15.
3. Girard P, Meyer G, Parent F, Mismetti P. Medical literature, vena cava filters and evidence of efficacy. A descriptive review. Thromb Haemost. 2014;111(4):761–9.
4. Kahn SR, Comerota AJ, Cushman M, et al. The postthrombotic syndrome: evidence-based prevention, diagnosis, and treatment strategies: a scientific statement from the American Heart Association. Circulation. 2014;130(18):1636–61.
5. Lee MJ, Valenti D, de Gregorio MA, Minocha J, Rimon U, Pellerin O. The CIRSE retrievable IVC filter registry:retrieval success rates in practice. Cardiovasc Intervent Radiol. 2015;38(6):1502–7.
6. Mismetti P, Laporte S, Pellerin O, et al. Effect of a retrievable inferior vena cava filter plus anticoagulation vs anticoagulation alone on risk of recurrent pulmonary embolism: a randomized clinical trial. JAMA. 2015;313(16):1627–35.
7. Muriel A, Jimenez D, Aujesky D, et al. Survival effects of inferior vena cava filter in patients with acute symptomatic venous thromboembolism and a significant bleeding risk. J Am Coll Cardiol. 2014;63(16):1675–83.
8. Prandoni P, Lensing AW, Prins MH, et al. Below-knee elastic compression stockings to prevent the post-thrombotic syndrome: a randomized, controlled trial. Ann Intern Med. 2004;141(4):249–56.
9. Prasad V, Rho J, Cifu A. The inferior vena cava filter: how could a medical device be so well accepted without any evidence of efficacy? JAMA Intern Med. 2013;173(7):493–5.
10. PREPIC Study Group. Eight-year follow-up of patients with permanent vena cava filters in the prevention of pulmonary embolism: the PREPIC (prevention du Risque d'Embolie Pulmonaire par interruption cave) randomized study. Circulation. 2005;112(3):416–22.
11. Ryan E, Kok HK, Lee MJ. Retrievable IVC filters: friend or foe. Surgeon. 2016. pii: S1479-666X(16)30051-8. doi: 10.1016/j.surge.2016.07.003.
12. Stein PD, Matta F. Vena cava filters in unstable elderly patients with acute pulmonary embolism. Am J Med. 2014;127(3):222–5.
13. Stein PD, Matta F, Keyes DC, Willyerd GL. Impact of vena cava filters on in-hospital case fatality rate from pulmonary embolism. Am J Med. 2012;125(5):478–84.

Venous Thromboembolism and DVT Thrombolysis/Thrombectomy

10

Michael Lee

10.1 Introduction

- The incidence of DVT in the general population is around 5 per 10,000 per annum (1 in 2000) and an additional 1 to 2 per 10,000 will have a new DVT combined with pulmonary embolism. The incidence is strongly age related in the population and is comparable in men and women.
- There are some factors, which increase the risk of DVT within subgroups of the general population.
  a. These include institutionalization with an 8-fold increase, which rises to 22 fold if accompanied by surgery.
  b. Trauma is associated with a 13-fold increase and malignancy with a 5-fold increase in risk.
  c. Women using the oral contraceptive pill or hormone replacement therapy have around a 2–4 fold increase.
  d. Inherited or acquired thrombophilia also increases the rise substantially

10.2 Natural History of DVT

- The natural history of DVT is that thrombus usually begins in the calf often in the cusp of a venous valve. A platelet cluster builds and grows towards the center with alternating layers of fibrin and red cells trapped between the layers of platelets.
- The thrombus initiates an inflammatory response from the endothelium leading to organization and eventual endothelialisation causes clot retraction.

M. Lee
Department of Radiology, Beaumont Hospital and Royal College of Surgeons in Ireland, Dublin, Ireland
e-mail: mlee@rcsi.ie

H.K. Kok et al. (eds.), *Interventional Radiology for Medical Students*,
DOI 10.1007/978-3-319-53853-2_10

- Retraction and organisation eventually leads to recanalisation and endothelialisation.
- Retraction occurs between 5 and 10 days, but during this time period embolisation of the thrombus to the pulmonary arteries can occur. Embolisation is more common with thrombus above the knee than below the knee.
- The retraction and recanalisation process often leads to destruction of the venous valves, which can lead to post thrombotic syndrome.

10.3 Post Thrombotic Syndrome

- After an acute DVT, up to 50% of patients develop post thrombotic syndrome (PTS) and 3–10% of these will have severe PTS. In particular, up to 75% of patients with iliofemoral DVT treated by anticoagulation alone will have chronic painful oedema and 40% will develop venous claudication.
- PTS is characterised by pain, swelling, heaviness, fatigue, itching, paraesthesia and venous claudication.
- Clinical signs of PTS include: oedema, venous ectasia, varicose veins, erythema, cyanosis, hyperpigmentation, lipodermatosclerosis and ulceration.
- Risk factors for PTS include residual thrombus in the first 3–4 weeks after a DVT, residual venous symptoms and signs at 1-month post DVT. Sub-therapeutic Warfarin therapy, recurrent DVT, thrombophilia and iliofemoral DVT treated by anticoagulation alone.
- PTS decreases quality of life and affects productivity. Over two million work days are lost annually in the US from leg ulcers and physical QOL in PTS is worse than QOL for osteoarthritis, angina and chronic lung disease.
- Current therapies for acute DVT are not thrombolytic, in other words, anticoagulation does not break up clot already formed. The goal of anticoagulant therapy is the prevention of pulmonary embolus, recurrent DVT and the prevention of thrombus propagation.
- Theoretically, techniques that dissolve or remove thrombus may prevent venous valve destruction and prevent PTS. Evidence is accruing to support this theory.

10.4 Methods of Thrombus Removal

- *Catheter Directed Thrombolysis*. The popliteal vein is accessed under ultrasound guidance and a long multi-sidehole infusion catheter is inserted from the popliteal vein to the iliac vein, recombinant tissue plasminogen inhibitor (r-tPA, alteplase) is infused as a 5–10 mg bolus and as a 1–2 mg per hour infusion over night. Studies have shown that complete lysis and venous patency is higher after catheter directed lysis. PTS and leg ulceration is significantly reduced, but bleeding complications are more common including intracranial haemorrhage.

- *Mechanical thrombectomy or pharmacomechanical thrombectomy.* Mechanical thrombectomy refers to thrombus removal using a device that either aspirates, macerates or vacuums clot. Many such devices are on the market. Pharmacomechanical thrombectomy refers to a mechanical device that is used in conjunction with a thrombolytic drug, commonly r-tPA.
- Pharmacomechanical thrombectomy costs less than catheter directed thrombolysis, can be performed in a single session in almost 80% of patients and does not have the same bleeding complications. Therefore there has been a move towards pharmacomechanical thrombectomy.
- It is important to realize that these therapies are performed in conjunction with standard anti-coagulation therapy.

10.5 Indications

- Currently, the main indication is patients with acute iliofemoral DVT (within 14 days), which has the highest incidence of PTS.
- An NIH study called the ATTRACT Trial has been recruiting for the last 4 years and will be reporting in 2017. The ATTRACT Trial will compare pharmacomechanical thrombectomy and anti-coagulation versus anti-coagulation alone for patients with both iliofemoral DVT and femoral DVT alone. The results of this trial are eagerly anticipated.

10.6 Contraindications

1. DVT that is more than 14 days old
2. Septicemia

10.7 Patient Preparation

- Patients should be fasting from midnight of the previous day.
- An IVC filter should be placed in selected patients before pharmacomechanical thrombectomy to prevent pulmonary embolism.
- Anti-coagulation should not be stopped for the procedure.

10.8 Procedure Description

- An IVC filter is first placed from a jugular route.
- Ultrasound-guided puncture of the popliteal vein if the thrombus is present from the iliac vein to the knee or the femoral vein is punctured if the clot is limited to the iliac segment. Contrast material is injected through an inserted sheath to document the extent of the thrombus.

- The device to be used is inserted and a number of passes made, usually with r-tPA also infused.
- The thrombus is completely removed usually within 2–3 h.
- Any residual stenosis in the iliac vein is stented with a venous stent (14–16 mm). A vascular sheath is left in situ and a further venogram performed the next day to ensure complete thrombus removal.

10.9 Complications

- Local complications such as bleeding at the puncture site are generally rare as this is a venous puncture in a low pressure system as apposed to an arterial puncture.
- Pulmonary embolus is also rare and the incidence is almost negligible with an IVC filter in place.
- Spontaneous bleeding complications are more common with catheter directed thrombolysis alone and much less common with pharmacomechanical thrombectomy.

Case

A 24-year-old woman on the oral contraceptive pill presented with sudden onset of dyspnoea and pleuritic chest pain. CT pulmonary angiogram confirmed a saddle pulmonary embolus with extension into both main pulmonary arteries. She was started on heparin and because she was also complaining of right groin pain, a duplex US was performed. Duplex US confirmed an above knee DVT extending into the iliac vein and lower IVC (Fig. 10.1).

Fig. 10.1 (**a**) CTPA showing saddle pulmonary embolus (*arrows*). (**b**) Because of the extensive thrombus extending into the IVC, it was decided to perform DVT pharmacomechanical thrombectomy. The image shows an injection of contrast material into the IVC after placement of a retrievable filter. Note the abrupt cut-off of the lower IVC because of thrombus filling the lumen (*arrows*). (**c**) Under US guidance, the popliteal vein was accessed and a sheath inserted. Through this an AngioJet thrombectomy device (Boston Scientific, Galway, Ireland) was used in conjunction with r-tPA to remove the clot from the leg and IVC. The image above shows an initial injection confirming clot within the femoral vein (*arrows*). (**d**) After a number of passes with the AngioJet thrombectomy device, the entire clot was removed. The IVC filter was removed at a later date

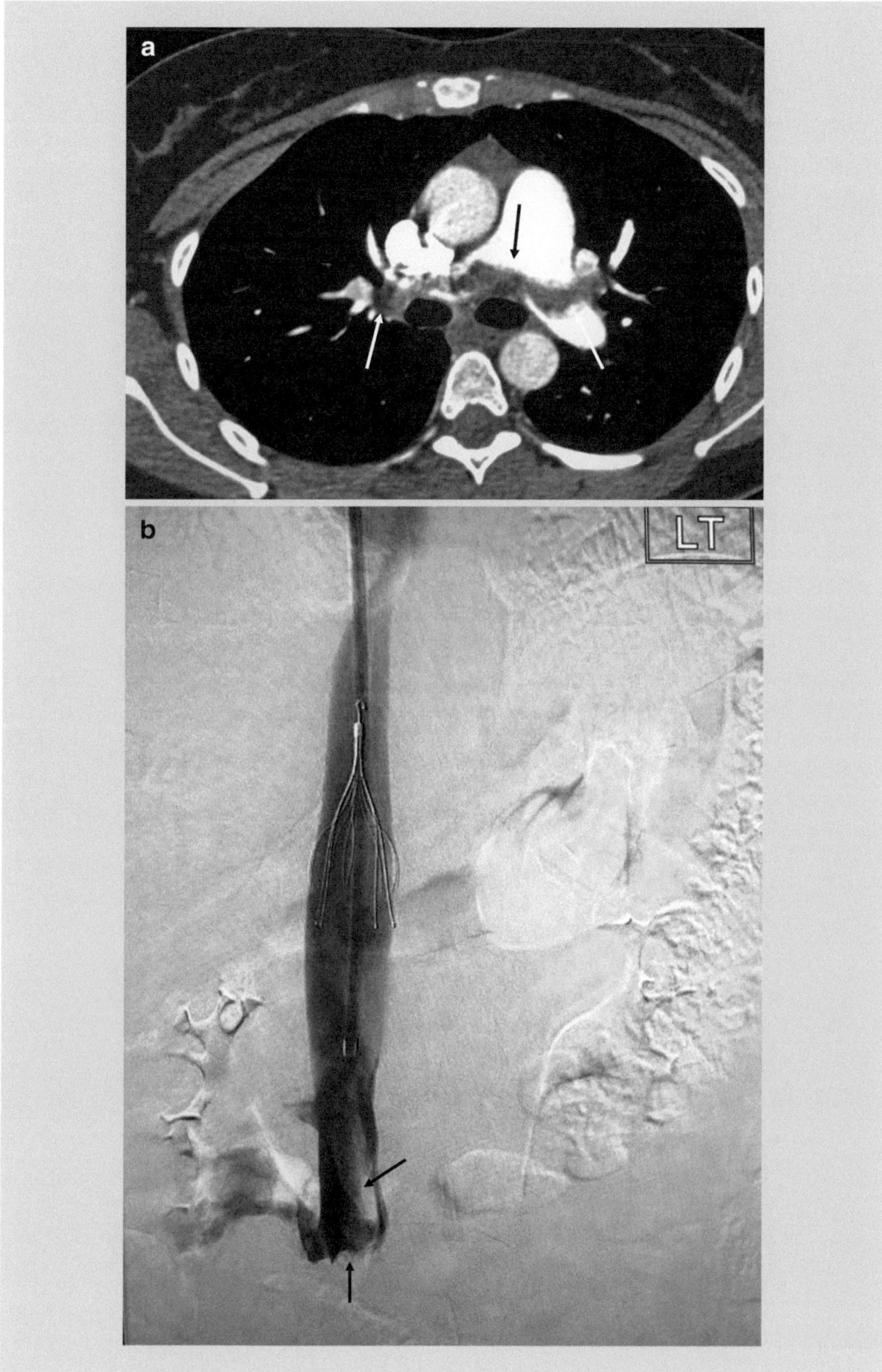
a
b
LT

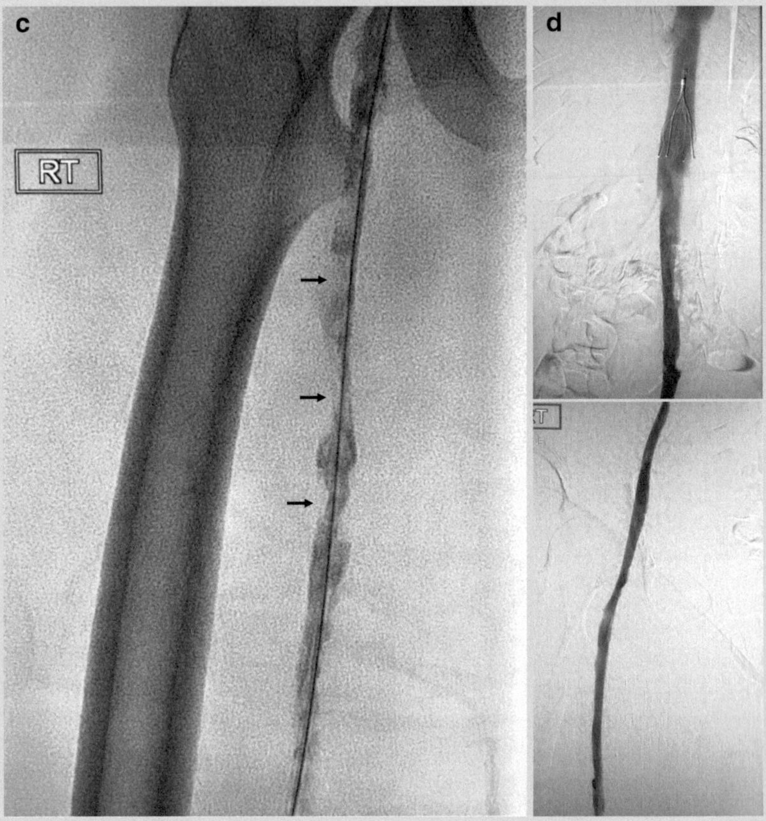

Fig. 10.1 (continued)

Key Points

- DVT can be associated with Post-Thrombotic Syndrome in up to 50% of patients.
- PTS occurs in up to 75% of patients with ilio-femoral DVT treated by anticoagulation alone and can be severe.
- Thrombus can be removed either by catheter directed thrombolysis using t-tPA, but at an increased risk of bleeding complications.
- Pharmacomechanical thrombectomy using a combination of low dose r-tPA and a mechanical device is now favoured for thrombus removal.
- Thrombus removal techniques should be confined to patients with ileo-femoral deep venous thrombosis or IVC thrombosis.

Suggested Reading

1. Fowkes FJI, Price JF, Fowkes FTR. Incidence of diagnosed deep vein thrombosis in the general population: systematic review. Eur J Vasc Endovasc Surg. 2003;25:1–5.
2. Haig Y, Enden T, Grøtta O, Kløw NE, Slagsvold CE, Ghanima W, Sandvik L, Hafsahl G, Holme PA, Holmen LO, Njaaastad AM, Sandbæk G, Sandset PM, CaVenT Study Group. Post-thrombotic syndrome after catheter-directed thrombolysis for deep vein thrombosis (CaVenT): 5-year follow-up results of an open-label, randomised controlled trial. Lancet Haematol. 2016;3(2):e64–71.
3. Kahn SR, Shrier I, Julian JA, et al. Determinants and time course of the postthrombotic syndrome after acute deep venous thrombosis. Ann Intern Med. 2008;149:698–707, 3. Post-thrombotic syndrome after catheter-directed thrombolysis for deep vein thrombosis (CaVenT): 5-year follow-up results of an open-label, randomised controlled trial.
4. Vedantham S, Goldhaber SZ, Kahn SR, et al. Rationale and design of the ATTRACT study: a multicenter randomized trial to evaluate pharmacomechanical catheter-directed thrombolysis for the preven- tion of postthrombotic syndrome in patients with proximal deep vein thrombosis. Am Heart J. 2013;165:523–30. [e523] 2.

Transjugular Intrahepatic Portosystemic Shunt (TIPS)

11

Hong Kuan Kok

11.1 Introduction

- Portal hypertension results from increased resistance to portal venous flow in patients with chronic liver disease and cirrhosis. Clinical manifestations of portal hypertension include ascites and gastro-oesophageal varices. Patients may also present with hepatic encephalopathy.
- The first line of management for ascites in chronic liver disease consists of medical therapy including diuretics (e.g. spironolactone) and dietary salt restriction followed by large volume paracentesis if conservative measures alone are unsuccessful.
- Management of gastro-oesophageal varices on the other hand is directed at reducing risk of bleeding and this is accomplished through the use of beta-blockers (e.g. propanolol) and prophylactic endoscopic banding of varices.
- In patients presenting with acute variceal haemorrhage, emergency resuscitation, urgent endoscopic ligation and use of vasoactive agents such as terlipressin or octreotide are the mainstay of initial management. Occasionally, local tamponade of the varices using a Sengstaken-Blakemore tube may be required pending more definitive management.
- TIPS is a complementary, minimally invasive procedure performed to reduce portal venous pressures and involves the creation of an artificial shunt between the portal and systemic venous circulation (portosystemic shunt) in patients with portal hypertension. In particular, TIPS has a major role to play in the treatment of refractory ascites or hydrothroax, where medical therapy has failed and variceal haemorrhage, in both prophylactic and acute settings.

H.K. Kok
Department of Radiology, Beaumont Hospital and Royal College of Surgeons in Ireland, Dublin, Ireland
e-mail: terrykok@gmail.com

H.K. Kok et al. (eds.), *Interventional Radiology for Medical Students*,
DOI 10.1007/978-3-319-53853-2_11

11.2 Indications

- Prophylaxis for recurrent variceal haemorrhage
- Bleeding gastric varices which are difficult to treat endoscopically
- Acute refractory variceal haemorrhage, not responding to medical or endoscopic therapy
- Refractory ascites or hepatic hydrothorax
- Hepatorenal or hepatopulmonary syndrome
- Portal hypertensive gastropathy
- Budd-Chiari syndrome

11.3 Contraindications

- Severe uncorrectable systemic coagulopathy
- Sepsis
- Severe right heart failure – the increased venous return to the right heart from the portosystemic shunt can precipitate cardiac decompensation
- Advanced hepatic encephalopathy – transient encephalopathy is common following TIPS and could worsen pre-existing encephalopathy
- Advanced liver failure as measured by Model for End-stage Liver Disease (MELD) or Child-Pugh scores, predicting poorer outcomes following TIPS
- Extensive portal vein thrombosis

11.4 Patient Preparation

- Comprehensive review of symptoms, signs, investigations and imaging with input from referring clinicians, hepatology services and interventional radiology.
- Typically performed as an inpatient procedure, either acutely or electively depending on the clinical context. Most cases are performed under general anaesthesia as this can be a long and painful procedure taking 2–3 h to complete.
- Fasting for at least 6 hours prior to the procedure, with anaesthetics pre-operative review as appropriate.
- Intravenous access, ideally at least 18 gauge for IV fluid infusion, sedation and resuscitation measures.
- Blood investigations including a contemporaneous full blood count, renal function tests and coagulation studies. Most operators would use a cut-off international normalised ratio (INR) of less than 1.5 and platelet count of greater than 50,000.
- Systemic coagulopathy and thrombocytopaenia which is not infrequently seen in patients with chronic liver disease will need particular attention and management prior to the procedure.

11.5 Procedure

- The right internal jugular vein is accessed under ultrasound guidance using the Seldinger technique. A long 10 French vascular sheath is placed over a guidewire and the tip is positioned in the IVC.
- Using an angled tip angiographic catheter, a branch of the hepatic vein (usually middle or right) is catheterised. A curved TIPS needle is then advanced through the liver parenchyma to cannulate a branch of the portal vein, creating an intrahepatic tract (Fig. 11.1a and 11.3).
- Pressure measurements are taken within the systemic and portal venous systems to calculate a mean portosystemic pressure gradient.
- A TIPS covered stent-graft is then deployed across the tract created between the hepatic (systemic) and portal veins. The stent has an uncovered portion that sits in the portal vein to allow continued flow from the portal vein to the liver (Fig. 11.1b and 11.3c).
- The stent is dilated with an angioplasty balloon to achieve the desired mean portosystemic pressure gradient reduction of <12 mmHg.
- Any varices which have bled can be embolised during the TIPS procedure.
- Haemostasis is achieved at the jugular puncture site with manual compression.

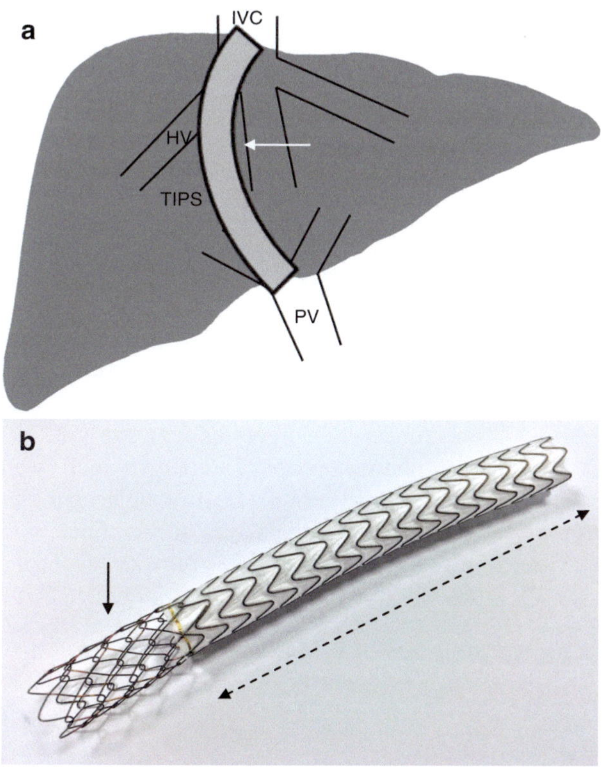

Fig. 11.1 (**a**) Diagram of the TIPS procedure showing placement of a TIPS stent graft (*arrow*) between the right hepatic vein (HV) and right portal vein branch (PV). (**b**) Typical TIPS stent-graft (Gore Viatorr) with a short uncovered portion (*solid arrow*) which is deployed in the portal vein and longer PTFE covered portion (*dashed arrow*) which is deployed across the intrahepatic tract and hepatic vein

11.6 Results

- TIPS is highly effective in reducing the incidence of variceal rebleeding when compared to endoscopic therapy (18% versus 66% at 2 years).
- Better control of refractory ascites compared to large volume paracentesis and may convert diuretic-resistant ascites to diuretic-sensitive ascites.
- May improve renal function in patients with hepatorenal syndrome.
- Effective in treating acute refractory variceal haemorrhage and should be performed in preference to surgery.
- The use of covered TIPS stent-grafts has resulted in good patency rates of 70–80% at 2 years.

11.7 Complications

- Mortality (1.7%) as a result of vascular or visceral perforation
- Encephalopathy (up to 30%, usually transient and mild)
- Haemorrhage
- Right heart failure from volume overload
- Stent-graft stenosis or occlusion (15–20% at 1 year requiring long term surveillance) (Case 11.2 and Fig 11.4)
- Infection of the implanted stent-graft

11.8 Case Examples

Case 11.1

A 45 year old man with cirrhosis and portal hypertension secondary to chronic alcoholic liver disease presents to the Emergency Department with a large variceal bleed. He was hypotensive and tachycardic at presentation with a haemoglobin level of 6 g/dl. His renal function and coagulation profile were normal and his MELD score was 8. He was resuscitated with fluid and blood products and underwent urgent upper gastrointestinal endoscopy which confirmed multiple oesophageal varices which were banded and injected (Fig. 11.2). Two days into his admission, he experienced a second episode of variceal haemorrhage which was successfully managed endoscopically. In view of these recurrent episodes of variceal haemorrhage, he underwent a TIPS procedure to minimise risk of future bleeding (Fig. 11.3).

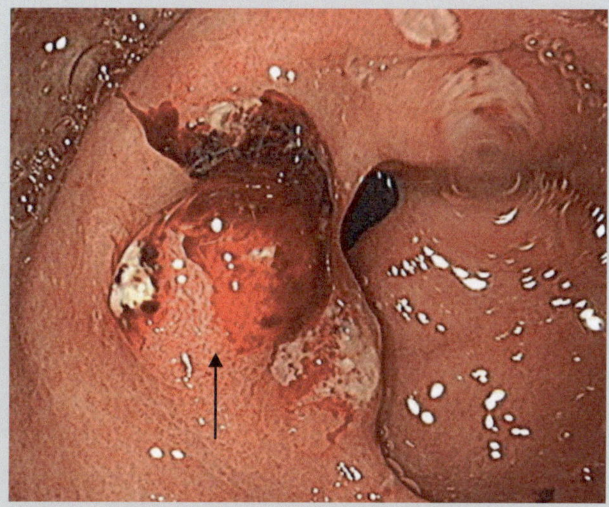

Fig. 11.2 Actively bleeding gastro-oesophageal varices (*arrow*) seen during the initial upper gastrointestinal endoscopy which were banded

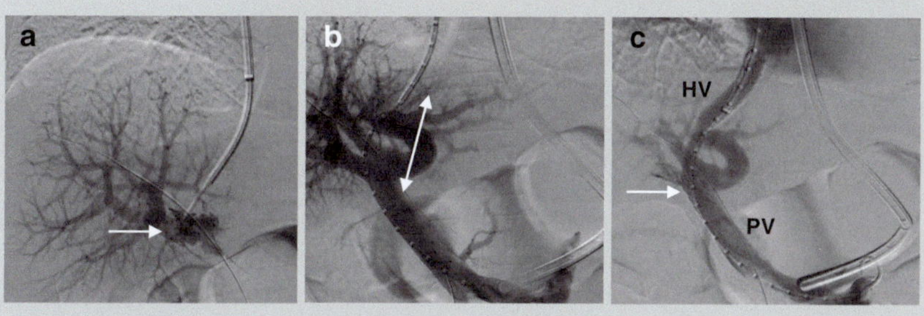

Fig. 11.3 (**a**) A vascular sheath and curved needle is passed via the jugular and middle hepatic vein into the right portal vein which is opacified with contrast material (*arrow*). (**b**) Following this, the intrahepatic tract (*arrow*) is measured and dilated. (**c**) A TIPS stent-graft is placed and a venogram shows direct flow of contrast from the portal vein (PV) across the stent (*arrow*) into the hepatic vein (HV), inferior vena cava and right atrium (portosystemic shunting)

Case 11.2

A 58 year old man who previously underwent TIPS presented with an acute variceal haemorrhage. Multiple large varices were seen at endoscopy and an ultrasound study showed absence of blood flow within the TIPS stent. He was brought to the Interventional Radiology suite for a portal venogram and further assessment (Fig. 11.4).

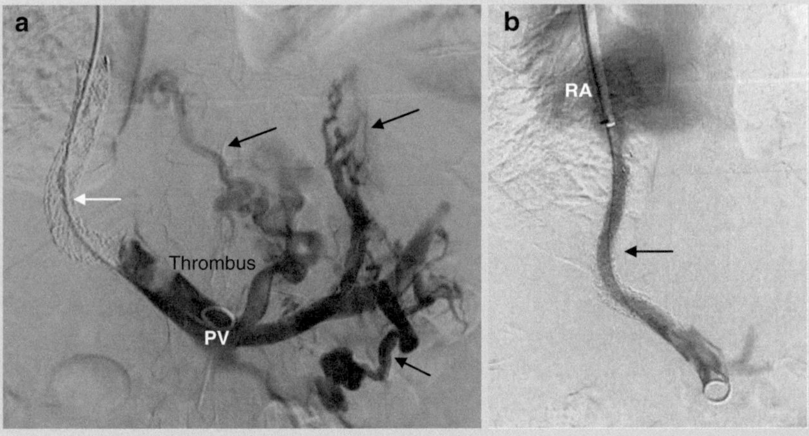

Fig. 11.4 (**a**) A catheter has been passed via the right internal jugular vein through the TIPS stent into the portal vein (PV). Contrast injection shows a filling defect consistent with thrombus within the portal vein and absence of flow through the TIPS stent confirming occlusion (*white arrow*). Multiple tortuous varices (*black arrows*) are seen surrounding the stomach and gastrooesophageal junction secondary to underlying portal hypertension and are responsible for the patient's acute presentation. (**b**) The TIPS stent (*arrow*) was successfully recanalised and the final venogram showed hepatopetal flow in the portal vein towards the right atrium (RA) with no residual flow within the varices

11.9 Post-procedure Care and Review

- Observation of vital signs and access site for local complications.
- Monitor for new or worsening encephalopathy. This is usually transient but may require adjunctive medical therapy with protein-restriction diets, lactulose, antibiotics and correction of biochemical and electrolyte abnormalities.
- Refractory severe encephalopathy may require reduction of the TIPS shunt using endovascular techniques to narrow the maximum diameter of the stent.
- Follow-up in accordance to local practice, typically with a baseline ultrasound study following the TIPS procedure and at 3–6 monthly intervals thereafter to monitor for development of stenosis or occlusion of the stent.

11.10 Discussion

- TIPS is an effective and minimally invasive procedure for the treatment of complications secondary to portal hypertension, most commonly variceal haemorrhage and refractory ascites.
- It involves creation of an intrahepatic shunt between a branch of the hepatic vein and portal vein followed by placement of a stent to maintain patency of the shunt tract, thereby reducing portal venous pressures.

- During the procedure, portal and systemic venous pressures are measured from the portal vein and right atrium respectively to calculate a portosystemic pressure gradient. This can be used to guide the degree of shunting required by limiting the maximum stent diameter during balloon dilatation. The target portosystemic pressure gradient is <12 mmHg.
- In contemporary practice, covered stent-grafts are placed as these devices have been shown to have superior patency rates (70–80% 2 year primary patency rates) over uncovered stents. However, regular imaging surveillance with ultrasound is required to detect complications such as stenosis and stent occlusion so that timely intervention can be performed.
- Embolisation of gastric and gastrooesophageal varices can also be performed during the TIPS procedure as further prophylaxis against future haemorrhage.
- Taking into account the significant medical co-morbidities and severity of underlying illness in patients with portal hypertension, TIPS procedures are performed in a relatively high-risk patient population. Complications from a TIPS procedure can range from transient encephalopathy (seen in up to 30%) to mortality from the procedure.

Key Points

- TIPS involves the creation of a portosystemic shunt in patients with portal hypertension. Common indications are acute variceal haemorrhage, prophylaxis against variceal rebleeding and refractory ascites.
- Hepatic encephalopathy is relatively common following TIPS and is usually transient.
- Patients require long-term clinical and imaging surveillance.

Further Reading

1. Kaufmann JA, Lee MJ. Vascular and Interventional Radiology: the Requisites. 2nd ed. Elsevier Saunders, Philadelphia. 2013.
2. Krajina A, Hulek P, Fejfar T, Valek V. Quality improvement guidelines for transjugular intrahepatic portosystemic shunt (TIPS). Cardiovasc Intervent Radiol. 2012;35:1295–300.
3. Pomier-Layrargues G, Villeneuve JP, Deschênes M, et al. Transjugular intrahepatic portosystemic shunt (TIPS) versus endoscopic variceal ligation in the prevention of variceal rebleeding in patients with cirrhosis: a randomised trial. Gut. 2001;48:390–6.

Percutaneous Renal and Ureteric Intervention

12

Elizabeth Ryan

12.1 Introduction

- Percutaneous urinary intervention is based upon needle and guidewire access to the urinary tract to facilitate decompression and stenting of obstruction from benign (e.g. renal or ureteric stones) or malignant disease.
- Open renal surgery for treatment of stone disease has now largely been replaced, with a significant associated reduction in morbidity.

12.2 Percutaneous Nephrostomy

Percutaneous access to the renal pelvi-caliceal system is performed with ultrasound or fluoroscopic guidance.

12.2.1 Indications

- Obstructive uropathy
- Urinary tract injury and urine leak
- Access for percutaneous urinary tract calculus treatment

E. Ryan
Department of Radiology, Beaumont Hospital and Royal College of Surgeons in Ireland, Dublin, Ireland
e-mail: lizryan1@gmail.com

H.K. Kok et al. (eds.), *Interventional Radiology for Medical Students*,
DOI 10.1007/978-3-319-53853-2_12

12.2.2 Contraindications

- Uncontrolled bleeding diathesis. International normalised ratio (INR) should be less than 1.5.
- Patient agitated or unable to lie in the lateral or prone position (usually due to respiratory compromise). This is a relative contraindication and may be managed by assistance from the Anaesthetic service.

12.2.3 Patient Preparation

- **Imaging** Review imaging to confirm the indication and assess the degree of dilatation.
- **Lab** Full blood count, coagulation status. International normalised ratio should be <1.5 and platelets >50 × 10^9/L.
- **Medications** Ideally clopidogrel/warfarin/novel anticoagulant medications would be stopped 5 days prior, but as this is usually an urgent or emergency procedure it is not typically feasible. Consult with Haematology to optimise coagulation status if necessary.
- **Antibiotics** Rapid life-threatening septic shock may follow percutaneous instrumentation in the setting of an obstructed infected pelvicaliceal system (known as a pyonephrosis). The patient should be adequately covered with appropriate intravenous antibiotics. Consult Microbiology for advice if necessary.
- **Fasting** Clear fluids are allowed up to 2 h pre-procedure; fasting for all other intake for at least 6–8 h.
- **IV access**
- **Written informed consent** should be documented after discussed of the procedure and its benefits, risks and alternatives.

12.2.4 Technique

- Prone or prone-oblique position ideally; lateral is possible but more difficult.
- Percutaneous passage of an access needle (18–22G depending on operator experience and preference) under image guidance. This is usually ultrasound-guided but may also be performed under fluoroscopy.
- When the needle tip enters the calyx, urine may be aspirated or may flow freely (indicating the system is under pressure).
- A small amount (5 ml or less) of iodinated contrast is injected to opacify the collecting system.
- A guidewire is passed through the access needle and curled in the renal pelvis, or ideally passed down the ureter if possible.
- 21/22G access needle: a microwire is advanced (0.014 inch), then a 3-piece trocar-dilator-sheath system (e.g. Accustick or Neff coaxial access system) is

passed over the microwire. This facilitates passage of a larger, more robust guidewire (0.035 inch), over which a nephrostomy may be placed.
- 18G access needle: proceed directly to placement of a standard 0.035 inch guidewire.
- The nephrostomy is a pigtail drainage catheter identical to those described previously (Image guided Drainage of Fluid Collections). The pigtail helps to secure its position. An external secure dressing (e.g. DrainFix) and/or suture can be sited for additional support.

12.2.5 Postprocedural Care

- Analgesia as required
- Bed rest for 2–4 h and regular monitoring of vital signs.
- Long-term nephrostomy catheters will require routine exchange. Consult with Interventional Radiology regarding appropriate frequency (typically every 3–6 months).

12.2.6 Complications

- Haemorrhage: blood-staining of the urine is common and usually clears within 2–3 days. Significant haemorrhage includes frank haematuria, large clots and haemorrhage within the parenchyma or outside the kidney and may require transfusion and/or intervention. (1–3%)
- Septic shock (1–3%)
- Injury to adjacent structure e.g. bowel, spleen (0.1–0.3%)
- Pneumothorax: associated with upper pole access via an intercostal route, and usually with large-calibre access tracts for percutaneous stone intervention (<0.1%)

12.3 Percutaneous Antegrade Ureteric Stent Placement

An alternative to external drainage via a percutaneous nephrostomy which is more comfortable and manageable for the patient when the requirement is medium- to long-term.

12.3.1 Indications

- Benign or malignant ureteric obstruction, including malignant tumours, ureteric strictures and retroperitoneal fibrosis.
- Prevention of ureteric obstruction by calculus fragments while undergoing lithotripsy for a renal calculus.
- Relief of ureteric calculus obstruction when definitive treatment is deferred to allow inflammation to settle.

12.3.2 Contraindications

- Acute pyonephrosis: priorities in the emergency setting include fast procedure time and minimal instrumentation of the acutely septic urinary tract. Stent placement may be performed several days after nephrostomy catheter placement when the acute phase has settled and the system has decompressed.
- Uncontrolled bleeding diathesis.

12.3.3 Patient Preparation

As for percutaneous nephrostomy placement.

12.3.4 Technique

- Prone or prone-oblique position.
- Percutaneous access as for percutaneous nephrostomy. If a nephrostomy is already sited, the locking pigtail should be released and a guidewire advanced into the pelvicaliceal system via the nephrostomy.
- The guidewire is advanced through the ureter into the bladder with the assistance of a catheter
- Antegrade stents are typically deployed over a guidewire and are pushed to an appropriate position with a specially-designed pusher. These are double pigtailed catheters (i.e. a pigtail at each end) which form their pigtails when the guidewire is retracted. Fluoroscopy allows visualisation of position throughout deployment.
- A "safety" nephrostomy may be left in-situ for several days if there is concern regarding haematuria and the risk of transient clot obstruction of the stent. This almost always resolves spontaneously within 2–3 days due to the lytic effect of endogenous urokinase. If a safety nephrostomy is sited, the patient should be pain-free with the nephrostomy clamped for 24 h prior to removal.

12.4 Percutaneous Nephrolithotomy (PCNL)

- This minimally invasive procedure has largely replaced open surgical nephrolithomy for the treatment of large renal calculi including staghorn calculi.
- Percutaneous access is as described above. The tract is dilated to a large calibre to facilitate stone/fragment extraction.
- An endoscope is used to visualise the calculus, which is fragmented using a Lithoclast or less commonly laser fragmentation.
- In most centres the procedure is performed in conjunction with a Urologist, who may require IR assistance for percutaneous access to the collecting system.
- Patient preparation, contraindications and post-procedural care are as described above for percutaneous nephrostomy placement.

- Complications are as described above. The risk of haemorrhage and pneumothorax are slightly increased due to the large calibre of the access tract but remain low (<5%).

Case

This patient presented with flank pain and CT demonstrated an obstructing calculus in the ureter with hydronephrosis. On discussion with Urology, it was decided to decompress the system via antegrade stent placement, and to perform a retrograde ureteroscopy for definitive stone treatment at a later date when acute inflammation has settled.

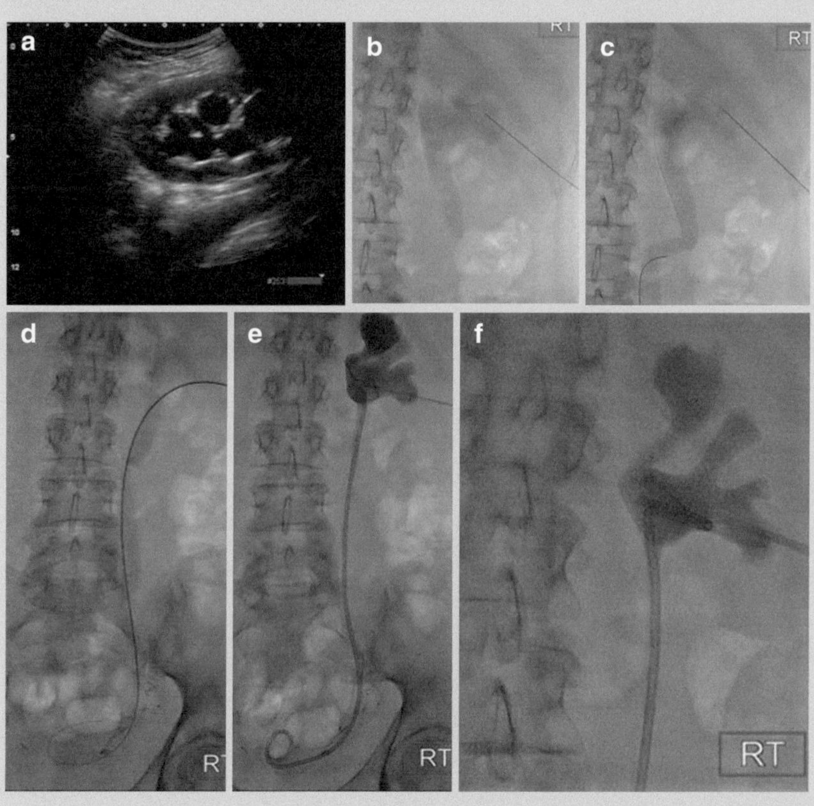

Nephrostomy and antegrade ureteric stent insertion. **(a)** A needle is inserted into a dilated lower pole calyx under ultrasound guidance. **(b)** Contrast is injected via the needle and fills the dilated pelvicaliceal system and ureter, down to the level of obstruction. **(c)** A guidewire is passed through the needle and it passes the ureteric obstruction. **(d)** A guidewire is passed to the urinary bladder and a sheath paased over the guidewire. **(e)** The stent is pushed over the wire and when the wire is retracted the pigtails from in the bladder and renal pelvis. **(f)** A nephrostomy tube is passed over the wire into the renal pelvis. After a day or two, if the patient remains well with the nephrostomy clamped it can be removed.

Key Points

- Percutaneous nephrostomy placement is used for relief of obstruction of the urinary tract due to benign and malignant disease.
- The percutaneous tract may be used to deploy a ureteric stent to bypass an obstruction.
- In the setting of large or staghorn renal calculus, a nephrostomy tract may be dilated to a large calibre to facilitate fragmentation and removal of the calculus. This is known as percutaneous nephrolithotomy.

Suggested Reading

1. Interventional Radiology. A survival guide. 4th ed. Kessel and Robertson. Elsevier; 2016.
2. Interventional Radiology Procedures in Biopsy and Drainage (Techniques in Interventional Radiology series) 2010. Gervais and Sabharwal (Editors). Lee and Watkinson (Series Editors). (Springer 2010).

Biliary and Gastrointestinal Intervention 13

Elizabeth Ryan

- Percutaneous intervention for biliary obstruction, sepsis and stone disease has been in existence since the advent of fine-bore needle access in the 1970s, and percutaneous cholecystostomy since the 1980s. These treatments have revolutionised biliary intervention, which formerly involved complex and often risky surgery.
- Decompression of biliary obstruction via percutaneous drainage may be life-saving in the setting of biliary sepsis, offering a bridge to definitive treatment of choledocholithiasis. Percutaneous stent placement for benign or malignant strictures offers relief of obstructive jaundice and its associated morbidity.
- Gastrointestinal tract intervention has traditionally been endoscopic or surgical, but there is a role for fluoroscopically-guided intervention in certain scenarios. Percutaneous gastrostomy placement (also known as Radiologically Inserted Gastrostomy or RIG) is an alternative to Percutaneous Endoscopic Gastrostomy (PEG).
- Gastrostomy tubes are indicated for long-term supplementation or replacement of oral feeding when oral intake is insufficient or contraindicated, for example due to neurological swallow impairment.
- The fluoroscopically-guided approach is particularly useful for patients with subtotal pharyngeal or oesophageal obstruction where passage of an endoscope is unfeasible or fails.
- Gastrointestinal tract stenting (Oesophageal tumors, obstructing colon tumours or gastric outlet obstruction) can be performed by endoscopists or Interventional Radiologists.

E. Ryan
Department of Radiology, Beaumont Hospital and Royal College of Surgeons in Ireland, Dublin, Ireland
e-mail: lizryan1@gmail.com

H.K. Kok et al. (eds.), *Interventional Radiology for Medical Students*,
DOI 10.1007/978-3-319-53853-2_13

13.1 Percutaneous Transhepatic Cholangiography (PTC)

- PTC is a technique used to access and image the biliary system. A needle is advanced through the abdominal wall and liver into a bile duct under ultrasound or fluoroscopic guidance. Contrast medium is then injected to fill the bile ducts, demonstrating the degree of dilatation and delineating the site of an obstruction or calculus. It also facilitates passage of a guidewire and catheter into the biliary tree for intervention.
- The advent of high quality cross-sectional imaging such as Magnetic Resonance Cholangiopancreatography (MRCP) has substantially reduced the role for primary diagnostic PTC and it is now usually reserved for patients requiring further biliary intervention or where non-invasive imaging is inconclusive.

13.1.1 Indications

- **Biliary Drainage**
  - Biliary obstruction due to benign or malignant strictures or choledocholithiasis.
  - Diversion of bile drainage in the setting of a bile leak (e.g. iatrogenic bile duct injury after laparoscopic choleystectomy).
  - Endoscopic retrograde cholangiopancreatography (ERCP) is the preferred access route to the biliary system. Transhepatic drainage is considered when ERCP is unfeasible (e.g. previous gastric surgery, anatomic variation) or unsuccessful.
  - Biliary drainage and stenting is also preferred for hilar obstructions when surgery is not feasible and where endoscopic drainage may not offer long term palliation.
- **Stenting**
  - Plastic stents are used for benign obstruction (strictures, calculi/sludge) and require routine 3 monthly change to prevent recurrent obstruction and biliary sepsis. Uncovered metallic stents cannot be removed and are reserved for malignant obstruction.
  - Plastic stents require a large transhepatic access tract (10 Fr) and are typically inserted and changed via ERCP. However, they can also be place transhepatically if required. Metal stents require a smaller access tract (6–9 Fr).

13.1.2 Contraindications

- **Uncontrolled bleeding diathesis** Patients with jaundice are predisposed to coagulopathy due to deranged liver function. Coagulation status should be measured and coagulopathy corrected prior to proceeding.
- **Gross ascites** Increases the risk of haemorrhage from the liver as the natural tamponade of the abdominal cavity wall is lost. Ascites can be drained prior to the procedure.

13.1.3 Patient Preparation

- **Imaging** should be reviewed prior to the procedure to confirm the indication and choose the appropriate site of access. The patient may need right and left lobes of the liver drained separately if there is a hilar lesion and sepsis. (It is often unnecessary to drain both in the absence of sepsis, as drainage of 25–30% of the liver is adequate to relieve jaundice).
- **Lab** Full blood count, coagulation status. International normalised ratio should be <1.5 and platelets >50 × 10^9/L, Group and Hold 2 units RCC
- **Medications** Clopidogrel/warfarin/novel anticoagulant medications should be held for a duration appropriate to the specific agent. Obstructed biliary sepsis is an emergency and it may be reasonable to proceed without waiting for clearance of anticoagulant medications. Given the coexistence of sepsis the risk of haemorrhage will be considerable increased and Haematology advice should be sought to optimise risk factors.
- **Antibiotics** Rapid life-threatening septic shock may follow percutaneous instrumentation in the setting of obstructed biliary sepsis. The patient should be adequately covered with appropriate intravenous antibiotics. Piperacillin/Tazobactam is the agent of choice because of high concentrations in bile and good gram positive and negative coverage
- **Fasting** Fasting for 8 h before the procedure. IV fluids are administered for 12 h before the procedure and for 24 h after the procedure
- **IV access**
- **Written informed consent** should be documented after discussed of the procedure and its benefits, risks and alternatives.

13.1.4 Technique

- Supine position.
- Right lobe access: mid-axillary line, 10th intercostal space. Left lobe access: epigastric region.
- Ultrasound guidance is typically used for left lobe access, either ultrasound or fluoroscopy may be used for right lobe access.
- An appropriate bile duct is punctured with a 21/22G needle and contrast is gently injected to outline the biliary tree.
- An 0.014/0.018 inch guidewire is advanced through the needle towards the central/hilar ducts. A co-axial trocar-introducer-sheath set is advanced over the guidewire, creating a larger access tract which allows passage of a more robust 0.035 inch guidewire and access sheath.
- A special catheter and hydrophilic guidewire may now be used to cross the obstructing lesion and down into the duodenum.

- **Catheter drainage:** a percutaneous drainage catheter may be sited and connected to an external drainage bag. Options include
  - a pigtailed drain left in the dilated ducts proximal to the obstruction called external drainage
  - an internal-external drain which passes through the obstruction into the duodenum. This has side-holes above and below the level of obstruction which facilitates drainage to the duodenum, but also allows bile to drain externally if internal drainage fails. This has a much more stable position and is less likely to inadvertently retract or displace.
- **Stenting:** a stent may be passed over the guidewire and opened at the level of obstruction. Pre- or post-dilatation may be performed with an angioplasty balloon if necessary.

13.1.5 Post-procedure Care

- Analgesia as required.
- Bed rest and frequent monitoring of vital signs for 4 h.

13.1.6 Complications

- Haemorrhage: arterial injury requiring management in 1–2% of cases
- Biliary leak ± peritonitis (<5%)
- Cholangitis (10–15%)

13.2 Percutaneous Cholecystostomy

- A percutaneous pigtail type drain may be sited within the gallbladder for drainage in certain clinical circumstances.
- The drain will need to remain in place until the process of healing has formed a tract around the drainage catheter, to prevent leakage of gallbladder contents into the abdominal cavity. This typically takes at least 4–6 weeks.

Indications: Cholecystostomy placement is reserved for

- Gallbladder empyema.
- Haemorrhagic cholecystitis and acalculous cholecystitis, typically in very ill patients with multi-organ dysfunction and diminished capacity to withstand acute sepsis.
- Elderly patients with acute cholecystitis who fail conservative management and in whom acute surgery is deemed to be "high-risk".
- Access for biliary drainage following failed ERCP and PTC (rarely required).

13.2.1 Contraindications

- Uncontrolled bleeding diathesis and large volume ascites are relative contraindications but can usually be treated to facilitate the procedure.

13.2.2 Patient Preparation

Patient preparation as for percutaneous biliary drainage. Additional considerations:

- This is often an emergency procedure and increased risk of haemorrhage with antiplatelet agents and NOACs may need to be accepted if delay is considered a greater risk to the patient.
- Consult Microbiology for advice regarding antibiotic cover for complicated cases - particularly for very ill patients with multi-organ dysfunction and multi-factorial acute illness (as is often the case for these procedures).
- Remember to advise the patient that the drain will remain in place for at least weeks 4–6 weeks. If the patient is medically fit for cholecystectomy the drain will remain in place until surgery.

13.2.3 Technique

- Supine position
- Ultrasound guidance for needle access to the gallbladder lumen.
- An inflamed gallbladder adherent to the anterior abdominal wall may be punctured directly. Alternatively, a transhepatic route is often advocated in order to reduce the risk of leakage into the peritoneum (a small leak around the tube will be contained between the gallbladder and liver).
- Once aspiration of contents confirms luminal placement of the needle tip, a stiff guidewire is advanced through the needle. The needle is removed leaving the wire in place and a pigtail drainage catheter is advanced over the guidewire and the tip curled within the gallbladder lumen.
- As for abscess drainage and indeed nephrostomy placement, pigtail catheters are available in a 3-piece trocar-stiffener-catheter tri-axial system which allows direct placement of the catheter under ultrasound guidance. This is an alternative to the multi-step technique described above. It is more prone to complication and is reserved for the experienced operator.
- The drainage catheter is secured with the locking pigtail and an external adhesive dressing ± a skin suture.

13.2.4 Post-procedural Care

- Bed rest for 4 h, regular monitoring of vital signs
- The drainage catheter should be flushed with saline and aspirated every 6–8 h to prevent blockage.
- Prior to removal the patient should have an asymptomatic trial of clamping of the catheter for at least 24 h, ideally 48 h.

13.2.5 Complications

- Catheter dislodgement/inadvertent removal (5%)
- Bile leakage and biliary peritonitis (<1%)
- Haemorrhage requiring transfusion or intervention (<1%)
- Bowel injury (<1%)

13.3 Percutaneous Gastrostomy Insertion

An alternative to a percutaneous endoscopic gastrostomy (PEG), this is inserted under fluoroscopic guidance without endoscopic guidance and is called a radiologically-inserted gastrostomy (RIG).

13.3.1 Indications

- Indicated for long-term feeding in the setting of mechanical or functional swallow impairment.
- Most commonly these are sited for patients with oropharyngeal tumours or neurological dysfunction.

13.3.2 Contraindications

- Uncontrolled bleeding diathesis.
- Patient condition or agitation precluding motion-free supine positioning or ability to maintain their respiratory status in the supine position. This is of particular relevance for some neurological or neurosurgical conditions. Airway support and general anaesthesia may be required.

- Gastrectomy or partial gastrectomy. Percutaneous options are available but are specialised and should be discussed with Interventional Radiology on an individual patient basis.

13.3.3 Patient Preparation

- **Imaging** Prior imaging should be reviewed prior to the procedure to assess for anatomical variance of relevance to the access tract.
- **Lab** Full blood count, coagulation status. International normalised ratio should be <1.5 and platelets >50 × 10^9/L.
- **Medications** Clopidogrel/warfarin/novel anticoagulant medications should be held for a duration appropriate to the specific agent.
- **Fasting** Fasting for at least 8 h before the procedure.
- **IV access**
- **Written informed consent** should be documented after discussed of the procedure and its benefits, risks and alternatives. Consent from next-of-kin may be necessary.
- **Nasogastric tube must be sited**

13.3.4 Technique

- Supine position
- Administer intravenous hyoscine butylbromide (Buscopan) to allow gastric relaxation. Note this may result in transient elevation of heart rate and should be limited or avoided in the setting of uncontrolled arrhythmia.
- The stomach is insufflated with room air via the nasogastric tube and the distended air-filled stomach is visualised with fluoroscopy.
- Gastropexy sutures (T-tacks/T-fasteners) are deployed to fix the anterior gastric wall against the anterior abdominal wall under fluoroscopic guidance. This is a short metal bar attached to a suture that is delivered through the skin into the gastric lumen via an access needle. The suture is pulled up to draw the stomach up to the abdominal wall and the suture is clamped at the skin to fix it. Typically, 3 or four point fixation is performed and the gastrostomy tract will be located at the centre point.
- The stomach is puncture with an 18 G needle and a stiff guidewire advanced. The tract is dilated and the length of the tract is measured.
- A gastrostomy is then inserted via a peel-away sheath and a balloon at the deep end of the gastrostomy is inflated with saline or water. Position is confirmed by contrast injection through the gastrostomy.

13.3.5 Post-procedure Care

- Bed rest for 4 h
- Regular monitoring of vital signs
- Remain nil-by-mouth (and per NG) for 24 h.
- If the patient is well and the abdomen is soft and non-tender at 24 h, clear fluid may be administered via the RIG. If this is well tolerated, RIG feeding can be introduced and the NG removed.
- Opinions differ regarding the removal of gastropexy sutures. Some advocate leaving the sutures for 2 weeks until the gastrostomy tract is formed. However, many cut them at 1–4 days post-procedure as they cause considerable discomfort and the gastrostomy balloon should be sufficient to maintain position.

13.3.6 Complications

- Peritonitis, usually due to dislodgement or inadvertent removal of the RIG. (<1%)
- Injury to adjacent structures (<1%)
- If the patient suffers from gastro-oesophageal reflux ± aspiration with RIG feeding, the RIG can be replaced with a gastrostomy with a jejunal extension.

13.4 Gastrointestinal Tract Stenting

13.4.1 Indications

- Relief of dysphagia in unresectable oesophageal carcinoma
- Temporary exclusion of oesophageal fistulae and perforations
- Gastric outlet or duodenal tumour obstruction
- Closed-loop colonic tumour obstruction

13.4.2 Contraindication

- No absolute contraindications.
- Patient condition including coagulation status should be optimised pre-procedure where possible.

13.4.3 Patient Preparation

- **Imaging** Assess prior imaging for planning of access and stent placement.
- **Lab** Full blood count, coagulation status. International normalised ratio should be <1.8 and platelets >50 × 10^9/L.
- **Medications** Clopidogrel/warfarin/novel anticoagulant medications should be held for a duration appropriate to the specific agent.
- **Fasting** Clear fluids are allowed up to 2 h pre-procedure; fasting for all other intake for at least 4 h.
- **IV access**
- **Written informed consent** should be documented after discussed of the procedure and its benefits, risks and alternatives.

13.4.4 Technique

- Supine for upper GI access, typical lateral decubitus for rectal access.
- The stricture is crossed with a guidewire and catheter, dilatation may be performed as appropriate, and a large 2–3 cm diameter metal stent is deployed under fluoroscopic guidance over a guidewire.
- Contrast injection confirms patency.

13.4.5 Post-procedure Care

- Bed rest for 4 h.
- Regular monitoring of vital signs.

13.4.6 Complications Occur in Approximately 10% of Patients and Include

- Perforation: perforation with a guidewire or catheter is usually without consequence but balloon dilatation or stent placement through a perforation is likely to require surgical management.
- Migration: covered stents are less prone to tumour ingrowth and occlusion but were traditionally more prone to migration. Newer covered stents have better anchoring and are less prone to migration.
- Sepsis

Case 13.1

This patient presented with right upper quadrant pain and jaundice with weight loss. MRCP demonstrated biliary dilatation due to an obstructing common bile duct tumour. ERCP failed to access the biliary tree from a retrograde approach.

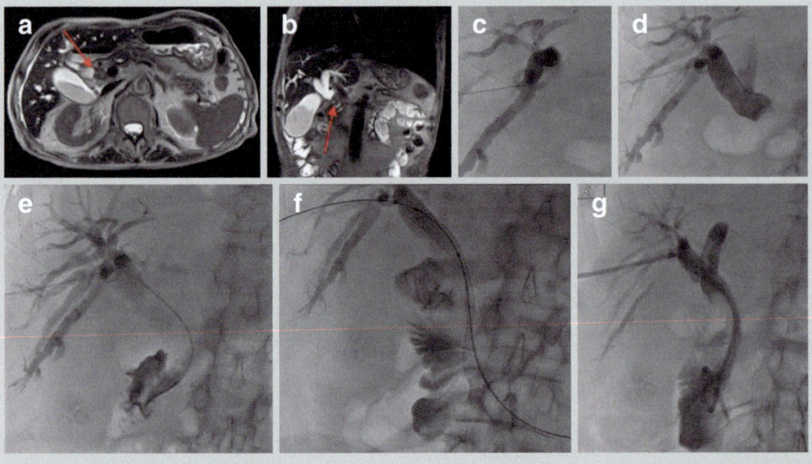

PTC and stent placement for biliary obstruction. (**a**) and (**b**) axial and coronal T2-weighted MRI shows dilated bile ducts and an obstructing tumour in the common bile duct (*arrows*). (**c**)–(**g**) PTC and stenting. Needle access to a right lobe bile and contrast injection fills the ducts (**c**), fallowed by passage of a guidewire to the point of obstruction (**d**). A catheter is advanced over the wire and the two are used together to negotiate through the obstruction (**e**). After a stiff guidewire is advanced to the distal duodenum, a stent is passed over the guidewire and opened across the obstructing tumour (**f**). Finally, an internal-external drain is left in as a security measure to ensure adequate drainage of bile (**g**). If the patient remains well, the drain can be removed and the percutaneous tract can be filled with embolic material to prevent haemorrhage and bile leak

Case 13.2

This patient has recurrent aspiration pneumonia due to impaired swallowing, on a background of motor neuron disease. He was referred for gastrostomy placement to facilitate continued enteral feeding without the need for a long-term nasogastric tube.

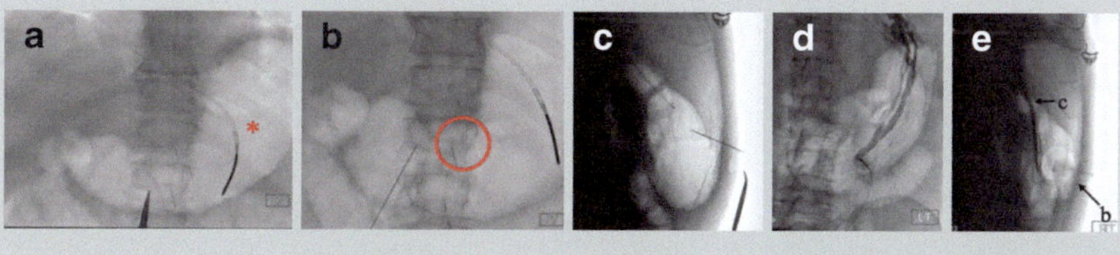

Radiologically-inserted gastrostomy. (**a**) The stomach is filled with air via a nasogastric tube (*) and the position of the gastric antrum is located by holding a metal object over the abdomen. (**b**) The stomach wall is affixed to the abdominal wall via 3 or 4 gastropexy sutures. In this image you can see the needle used to pass the suture through the abdominal wall and stomach wall into the gastric lumen. A tack that has already been deployed is seen within the *circle*. (**c**) A lateral view is helpful to confirm that the needle tip is in the gastric lumen, both for deployment of gastropexy sutures and for the needle access that will form the RIG tract. (**d**) After the tract is dilated and the gastrostomy is deployed, contrast is injected through it. You can see the contrast outlining the rugal folds of gastric mucosa which confirms intraluminal position. (**e**) A lateral view shows the contrast pooling at the posterior wall of the stomach (**c**) (remember the patient is lying supine) and additionally the anchoring balloon can be seen within the gastric lumen (**b**)

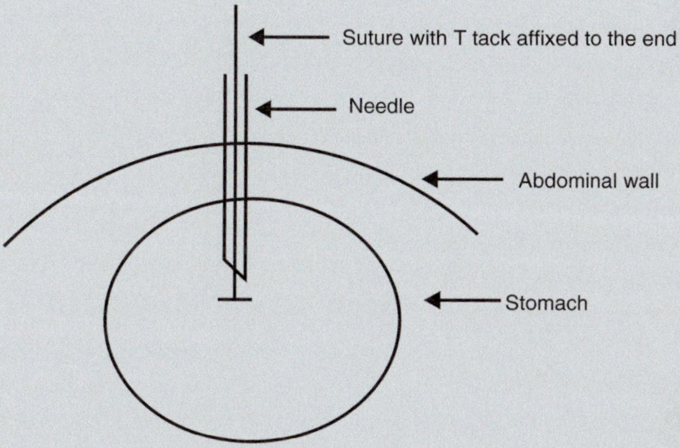

Schematic of gastropexy placement in a cross-sectional view

Key Points

- Percutaneous biliary drainage is a technique for imaging the biliary system and relief of biliary obstruction via drain placement or stenting.
- Percutaneous cholecystostomy placement is used for drainage of gallbladder empyema, haemorrhagic and acalculous cholecystitis and for patients unfit for surgery. The drain must remain in place until a tract has formed around it or until cholecystectomy is performed.

- Percutaneous gastrostomy placement under fluoroscopic guidance (RIG) is a useful alternative to endoscopic insertion. These are used for feeding when oral intake is insufficient or contraindicated.
- GI tract stents are placed for relief of obstruction and exclusion of fistulae and may be placed endoscopically or with fluoroscopic guidance.

Suggested Reading

1. Interventional Radiology. A survival guide. 4th ed. Kessel and Robertson. Elsevier; 2016.
2. Interventional Radiology Procedures in Biopsy and Drainage (Techniques in Interventional Radiology series) 2010. Gervais and Sabharwal (Editors). Lee and Watkinson (Series Editors). (Springer 2010).

Image Guided Biopsies

14

Timothy Murray and Michael Lee

14.1 Introduction

- Image guided biopsy is widely performed in all organ systems for tissue sampling, either of abnormal tissue that has been identified, or indiscriminate biopsy in cases of organ dysfunction to obtain representative tissue for histological diagnosis.
- The use of real-time image guidance allows targeted biopsy of even small lesions, and the avoidance of adjacent organs, vessels or collecting systems. The most commonly employed imaging modality is ultrasound, which is ideal for superficial organs like the thyroid, or solid organs such as the liver or kidneys. In addition, special ultrasound probes used transrectally, transvaginally, or endoscopically allow the biopsy of lesions within genitourinary, gastrointestinal and respiratory tracts.
- Ultrasound is limited by poor transmission of sound waves through air and bone however. CT gives excellent visualisation of structures within aerated lung, bone, and where loops of air-filled bowel are located. This permits biopsy of lung, bone or structures deep within the abdomen or pelvis. Fluoroscopy may also be used for bone biopsy.
- Other techniques such as MRI or PET guided biopsy are performed on occasion, however are limited by availability and cost.

T. Murray
Department of Radiology, Beaumont Hospital, Dublin, Ireland
e-mail: murraytim0@gmail.com

M. Lee (✉)
Department of Radiology, Beaumont Hospital and Royal College of Surgeons in Ireland, Dublin, Ireland

H.K. Kok et al. (eds.), *Interventional Radiology for Medical Students*,
DOI 10.1007/978-3-319-53853-2_14

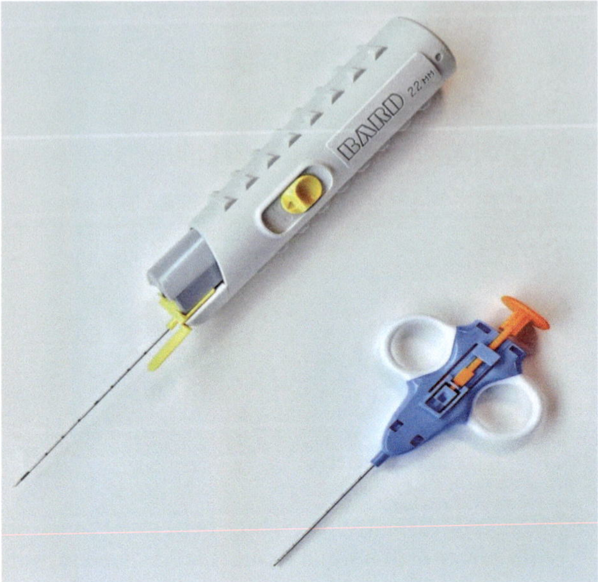

Fig. 14.1 Examples of commercial needles which are suitable for image-guided biopies. Most needle tips are visible on both CT and ultrasound. Where only fluid is required, such as to exclude infection or fine needle aspiration (FNA) for cytologic analysis, a standard needle of the appropriate length and gauge is used

- The risks of biopsy depend on systemic factors such as coagulopathy, and regional factors such as adjacent organs with can be inadvertently injured.
- In addition, certain specific malignant lesions carry a risk of seeding along the biopsy tract, such as osteosarcomas and certain salivary gland tumours. Where such lesions are within the differential diagnosis, biopsy should be planned in conjunction with the relevant oncological surgeon to ensure the biopsy tract will be included in any primary oncological resection, thus preventing the need for additional resection.
- Where multiple lesions exist, such as in cases of suspected metastatic malignancy, biopsy should target the lowest-risk area, such as superficial lymph nodes. Occasionally, dedifferentiated cytology within distant metastases may necessitate additional biopsies for definitive identification of the primary tumour.
- The size and number of biopsy cores required vary with organ and local practice. Biopsies of solid organs such as the liver and kidney are typically performed with 16–20 G core needles, with smaller gauge needles often requiring additional cores. Certain lesions such as in the parotid or thyroid may only require fine needle aspiration for diagnosis. Traditionally, a diagnosis of lymphoma required a surgical excision of a node, however there is increasing acceptance of image-guided biopsy in the first instance (Figs. 14.1 and 14.2).

14.2 Indication

- Investigation of organ dysfunction
- Biopsy of a mass lesion
- Biopsy of enlarged lymph nodes
- Sampling of infection for culture and sensitivity

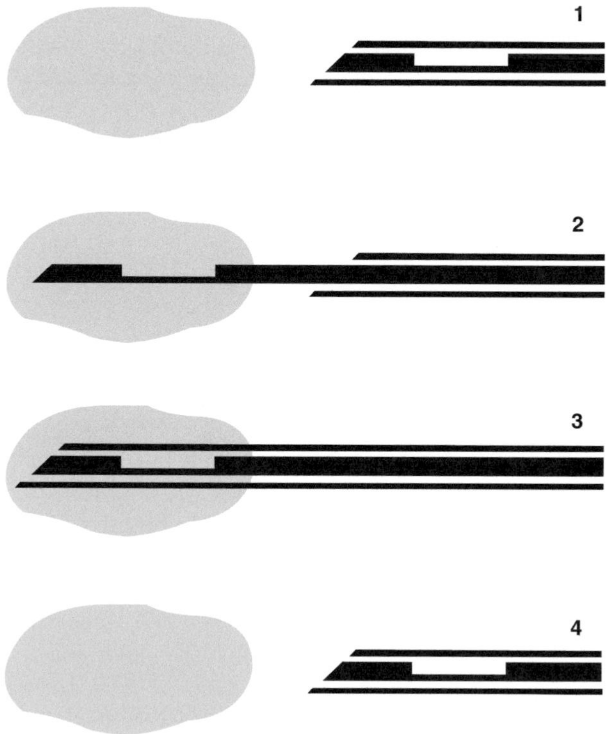

Fig. 14.2 Mechanism of a core biopsy gun. 1. Core biopsy needle advanced to lesion. 2. Needle inserted into lesion. 3. Outer sheath fired, cutting a core of tissue. 4. The entire biopsy needle is removed (Image used with written permission from BetterCare, Electronic Book Works, Cape Town, ZA)

14.3 Procedure Contraindications

- Coagulopathy (relative)
- Caution in approach where differential includes a tumour capable of seeding

14.4 Complications

- Haemorrhage or vascular injury (<6.6% depending on biopsy site)
- Visceral injury
- Injury to non-target viscera
- Tumor tract seeding (0–3.4%)
- Sedation reaction
- Anaphylaxis
- Death (1 in 3000 for liver biopsy)

14.5 Preparation

- Written informed consent
- Fasting (where sedation is required)
- Peripheral IV Access (where sedation is required)

- Enquire about anticoagulation and anti-platelet agent use.
- In locations where the risk of haemorrhage is moderate or high, or where there is underlying coagulopathy, coagulation screen and platelet levels should be performed in advance. For low-risk biopsies (superficial compressible structures) or in low-risk patients (outpatients without preexisting comorbidities), routine screening is not necessary. Suggested ranges as below:
  - INR <1.5 for high-risk (deep) biopsies such as intraabdominal or intrathoracic organs.
  - INR <2.0 for low-risk (superficial) biopsies such as superficial lymph nodes and thyroid.
  - Platelets >50,000/ml for high-risk biopsies, >25,000/ml for low-risk biopsies.
- IV heparin should be stopped 6–12 h prior and can be restarted after 12 h.
- Low-molecular weight heparin – Stop 12 h before and restart 12 h after procedure.
- Warfarin stopped 3–5 days, check INR prior to procedure, restart following procedure.
- Aspirin should only be withheld in high-risk biopsies. In these cases, it may be withheld for 5 days prior to procedure, and restarted following the procedure.
- Clopidogrel should be stopped 3–5 days prior to procedure following consultation with prescribing clinician (e.g. Cardiologist for coronary artery stents), restart following procedure.
- Dabigatran and other new oral anticoagulant medications should be stopped 1–2 days before the procedure if the creatinine clearance is <50 ml/min, stop 3–5 days if the creatinine clearance is >50 ml/min.
- Continuous hemodynamic monitoring where sedation is required, or in locations with a risk of bleeding or pneumothorax.

14.6 Technique (Overview)

14.6.1 Non-targeted Biopsy

- A representative area of organ parenchyma, such as the liver or kidney, is chosen, with care to avoid visible vessels or adjacent structures.
- Local anaesthesia is injected under guidance down to the level of the organ capsule where appropriate. Breath holding is employed as necessary if the organ is prone to movement with respiration. A biopsy device is inserted along the anaesthetised tract to the level of the desired parenchyma, which is then sampled.
- Following sampling, the area can be sonographically observed to assess for early complications such as haemorrhage.

14.6.2 Targeted Biopsy

- A discrete lesion, usually picked up on cross-sectional imaging, which requires sampling.
- The technique is essentially the same as a non-targeted biopsy, however greater emphasis is placed on positioning, and thus breath holding where appropriate. Ultrasound is most commonly employed, however CT or MRI can be used for challenging lesions.
- Care is taken when biopsying malignant lesions, as these often consist of friable and disorganised tissue which are more prone to haemorrhage. Where possible, the sampling needle should pass through a normal layer of the organ before entering the lesion. Theoretically, this should decrease the incidence of hemorrhage

14.7 Post-procedural Care

- Observation with regular monitoring of haemodynamic stability should be performed over 2–4 h post biopsies. Most procedural complications are evident by this time. There is little evidence to suggest any benefit to lying in the supine, prone or lateral position.

14.8 Specific Biopsies

14.8.1 Liver

- Liver biopsies are commonly performed. Non-targeted liver biopsies are performed in the investigation of liver disease, both to assess for the underlying cause and to establish the histological stage of the liver disease, which has prognostic and therapeutic implications.
- Targeted biopsies are performed for the investigation of focal lesions. The liver is a common site for metastasis at presentation. Primary liver lesions, whilst less common, can also be definitively characterised on histology. In cases where the biochemical and imaging findings are strongly suggestive of hepatocellular carcinoma in a cirrhotic liver, however, a liver biopsy may not be necessary and empiric treatment is often offered.
- Transjugular biopsy, performed via the internal jugular vein, is now rarely performed, often limited to uncorrectable coagulopathy. This resembles the initial steps of a TIPS procedure in terms of achieving hepatic venous access, at which time a transjugualar liver biopsy needle system is used to sample liver paren-

chyma. Specific complications in relation to liver biopsy include bile duct or gall bladder injury leading to the development of a biloma or biliary peritonitis. Non-target visceral injury includes pneumothorax or bowel perforation. Plugged liver biopsy can be performed in patients who require a biopsy but have a coagulopathy that is difficult to reverse. Patients receive platelets and fresh frozen plasma as required before and during the procedures and a co-axial approach is used. A 19 gauge needle is inserted to the target lesion and a 20 gauge core biopsy needle inserted through the 19 gauge needle to obtain tissue samples. When adequate tissue has been obtained, gelatin sponge (Gelfoam) plugs are inserted into the 19 gauge needle and pushed into the biopsy track as the needle is withdrawn. This serves to tamponade the biopsy track and minimise potential bleeding.

Case 14.1

- A 56 year old male is being worked up for a new diagnosis of colorectal cancer following discovery of a non-obstructing caecal mass on screening endoscopy. A staging CT of the thorax, abdomen and pelvis revealed a solitary lesion within the left lobe of liver which was concerning for a liver metastasis.
- Obtaining a biopsy for confirmation is required to guide further management for the patient including potential surgical and chemotherapeutic options (Fig. 14.3).

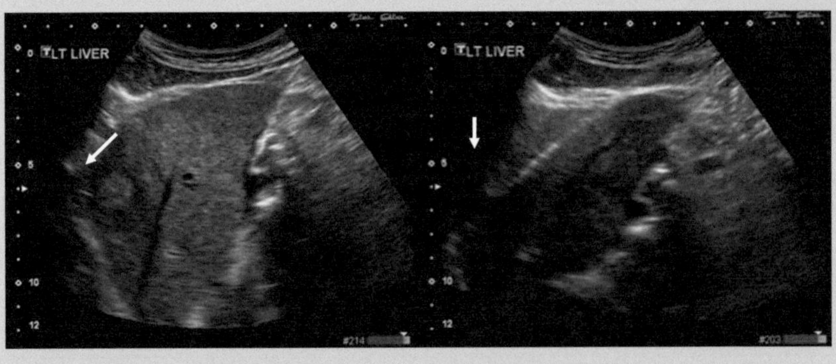

Fig. 14.3 Ultrasound demonstrates a hyperechoic lesion (*arrow*) within the left lobe of liver. Using real-time ultrasound guidance, a 20 G biopsy needle (*arrow*) is advanced to the level of the lesion, and several cores of tissue are obtained and placed in formalin for histological examination

14.8.2 Adrenal Biopsy

- Adrenal biopsy may be performed using CT or ultrasound, depending on the size and visibility of the lesion. The most common indication is for histological assessment of an adrenal lesion without characteristic appearance on CT/MR imaging. Patient preparation, contraindications, risks and post-procedural care are similar to that of liver biopsy. As expected, the risk of damage to the adjacent kidney should additionally be communicated, whilst the risk of liver damage is lower.

14.8.3 Kidney

- Renal biopsies are typically performed under ultrasound guidance. The most common indication is for further evaluation of suspected intrinsic renal disease (e.g. glomerulonephritis) or for assessment of a renal mass lesion (targeted). Patient preparation, contraindications, risks and post-procedural care resemble that of the above procedures, substituting the risk of renal collecting system injury in lieu of biliary injury.

14.8.4 Head and Neck

- Head and neck biopsies are commonly performed under ultrasound (superficial structures such as the thyroid, cervical nodes or superficial lobe of the parotid gland) or CT (deep structures such as the retropharyngeal space and the deep lobe of the parotid gland). The most common indication is for histopathologic assessment of a mass lesion. Specific risks include damage to important neuromuscular bundles within the head and neck including the facial nerve or the recurrent laryngeal nerve. Furthermore, haematoma formation in relation to the upper airway can cause airway compromise.

Case 14.2

- A 54 year old male presents with a 6 month history of intermittent bleeding from the left nostril and intermittent right frontal headaches. Flexible endoscopy reveals a mass deep to the posterior nasopharyngeal mucosa, with several areas of mucosal ulceration. An MRI is requested to assess for an underlying lesion.

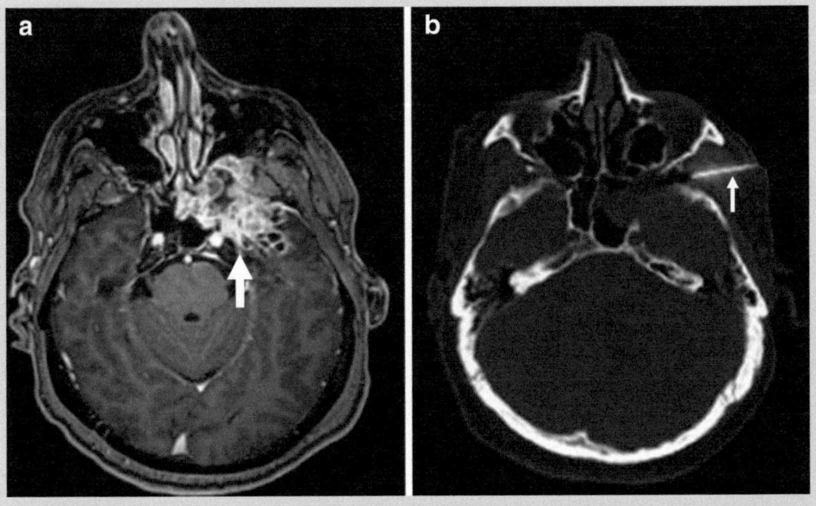

(**a**) Axial post-contrast fat-saturated T1-weighted MRI demonstrates a cystic enhancing lesion within the right pterygopalatine fossa invading posteriorly into the floor of the anterior cranial fossa (*thick arrow*). (**b**) CT-guided biopsy of the lesion was performed (*thin arrow*), with 22 G cores of tissue obtained and placed in formalin for histological examination.

14.8.5 Lung

- Lung biopsies are typically performed under CT guidance, however if a target lesion extends to the chest wall it may be suitable for ultrasound guided biopsy. Specific risks with lung biopsy are pneumothorax, pulmonary haemorrhage and air embolism. The rate of pneumothorax is 12–45%, with 2–15% requiring chest tube insertion. Following biopsy, patients and vital signs are monitored for 4 h. An erect chest radiograph is performed at 1–4 h (or sooner if the patient is symptomatic). If the patient remains well at 4 h and a visible pneumothorax has been excluded on the chest radiograph, the patient may be discharged with appropriate aftercare instructions.

14.8.6 Musculoskeletal

- The location of bone or soft tissue lesions determines the chosen modality, typically fluoroscopy or CT. Special considerations include injury to the adjacent neurovascular bundle and fracture. Consideration should be given to the potential for spinal cord damage with vertebral biopsy. The risk of tumour seeding is considered high in sarcomas, and any biopsy of a suspected primary bone malignancy should thus be performed only after appropriate multidisciplinary discussion. This allows the biopsy tract to be completely excised at subsequent surgery should the lesion require resection. Without this precaution, the surgeon may need to extend the operative field to excise the tract, and the removal of each tissue plane and muscle group can have profound implications on subsequent function when planning function-sparing amputations.

14.9 Results

Reported success rates with image-guided biopsy range from 70% to 90%, with overall mean success of 85%. Overall major complication rates should be below 2% regardless of organ.

Key Points

- Image-guided biopsy is a widely-used technique, which permits histological analysis of a range of lesions and organ disorders.
- The use of real-time image guidance reduces the risk of damage to the surrounding structures.
- The risk of complications is not eliminated however, and is typically specific to the organ in question and it's adjacent structures.
- Pre-procedural preparation and post-procedural care should be tailored to the risk of each biopsy. Low-risk procedures may be suitable for outpatient biopsy, while high-risk procedures may require pre-procedural optimisation and correction of coagulopathy, in addition to post-procedural observation.

Further Reading

1. Gupta S, Wallace MJ, Cardella JF, Kundu S, Miller DL, Rose SC. Quality improvement guidelines for percutaneous needle biopsy. J Vasc Interv Radiol. 2010;21(7):969–75.
2. Laurin, LP, Bonnardeaux, A, Leblanc, M, Dube, M. Percutaneous renal biopsy. INTECH Open Access Publisher; 2012.
3. Malloy PC, Grassi CJ, Kundu S, et al. Consensus guidelines for periprocedural management of coagulation status and hemostasis risk in percutaneous image-guided interventions. J Vasc Interv Radiol. 2009;20(7):S240–9.
4. Rockey DC, Caldwell SH, Goodman ZD, Nelson RC, Smith AD. Liver biopsy. Hepatology. 2009;49(3):1017–44.
5. Winokur RS, Pua BB, Sullivan BW, Madoff DC. Percutaneous lung biopsy: technique, efficacy, and complications. Semin Intervent Radiol. 2013;30(2):121–7.

15 Image Guided Drainage of Fluid Collections

Damien O'Neill and Hamed Asadi

15.1 Introduction

- A collection forms when fluid collects in a potential space. Fluid can be a transudate or an exudate determined by the biochemical composition. Collections can occur anywhere in the body. Patients may present with symptoms depending on the site of collection and its contents, e.g. shortness of breath, swelling, pain or discomfort.
- Treatment is determined by the severity of symptoms. The natural sequela of collections vary. They can resolve or an inflammatory process can ensue. The inflammatory response can result in focal inflammation with formation of suppurative exudate or abscess formation.
- Clinical manifestations of an abscess include general malaise, swinging pyrexia and SIRS (Systemic Inflammatory Response Syndrome). Initial treatment is with systemic intravenous antibiotics guided by organism sensitivity. However, many will not resolve until drained either radiologically or surgically.
- IR drainage is a minimally invasive alternative to surgery in many cases, provided the collection is visible by imaging and there is a safe access route to the abscess.

D. O'Neill, MRCS, MMedSc (✉)
Department of Radiology, Beaumont Hospital, Dublin, Ireland
e-mail: damienconeill@rcsi.ie

H. Asadi, MD, PhD, FRANZCR, CCINR, EBIR
Interventional Neuroradiology Service, Austin Health, Melbourne, Victoria, Australia

School of Medicine, Faculty of Health, Deakin University, Victoria, Australia
e-mail: hamed.asadi@austin.org.au

H.K. Kok et al. (eds.), *Interventional Radiology for Medical Students*,
DOI 10.1007/978-3-319-53853-2_15

- Abscess drainage by IR is generally called percutaneous abscess drainage (PAD) and is one of the most significant advances in patient care in the post-operative patient. Repeat abdominal surgery to drain a post-operative abscess is associated with an increased mortality and significant morbidity.
- Ultrasound or CT imaging are generally used to guide drainage. In certain circumstances intra-cavitary US can be utilised to gain access to sites, which may be inaccessible by the percutaneous route, such as endovaginal, endorectal.
- Ultrasound has an advantage over CT during placement because the position of the needle/catheter can be monitored in real-time. This is compared to CT where a stop and shoot technique is used, as the needle is advanced, repeat CT images are performed to check that the catheter is in the correct place.
- A sample is sent for laboratory analysis to determine the contents of the fluid depending on the clinical indication, which can include microbiology, biochemistry, cytology or histopathology.

15.2 Procedure Indications

- Infected collection/abscess
- Pleural or peritoneal fluid
- Joint effusion

15.3 Procedure Contraindications

- Bleeding diasthesis – relative
- Lack of safe access route
- Lack local expertise and experience

15.4 Patient Preparation

- Comprehensive review of symptoms, signs, investigations and imaging with input from referring clinicians and IR.
- Depending on the clinical condition of the patient, drainage can be performed as an outpatient e.g. seroma, however more commonly performed as an inpatient procedure due to clinical condition.
- Most cases are performed under local anaesthesia with some cases necessitating conscious sedation, for particularly sensitive sites or poorly co-operative patients.

- Blood investigations including a full blood count and coagulation studies should be performed.
- Most operators would use a cut-off international normalised ratio (INR) of less than 1.5 and platelet count of greater than 50,000 depending on the circumstances.
- If there is significant risk to witholding anticoagulation or bleeding diasthesis, then drainage can be attempted with a drainage system of smaller calibre.
- If the patient has elevated inflammatory indices and/or a fever, the patient should be commenced on IV antibiotics (after appropriate blood cultures have been obtained) before abscess drainage. PAD often causes a transient bacteraemia which requires antibiotic cover.

15.5 Complications

- Vascular or visceral perforation
- Haemorrhage
- Septic shower and sepsis

15.6 Equipment (Fig. 15.1)

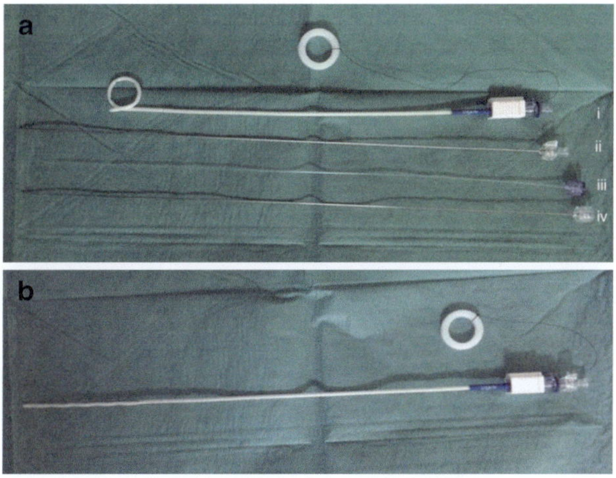

Fig. 15.1 (**a**) The typical contents of a drainage catheter set: *(i)* pigtail drain, *(ii)* inner metal stiffener, *(iii)* plastic stiffener and *(iv)* sharp metal trocar. The pigtail loop at the end of the drainage catheter helps to secure the catheter position within the abscess cavity. (**b**) Pigtail catheter straightened and placed over the metal stiffener ready for insertion over a guidewire

15.7 Case Study

Case 15.1

- US guided drainage of ascites was performed in a 45-year-old man with intra-abdominal fluid that was compromising his respiratory function. Initially an ultrasound scan of the abdomen is performed to confirm the presence of ascites and to identify the deepest pocket with a safe access route, avoiding major vascular bundles, e.g. inferior epigastric artery (Fig. 15.2).
- Local anaesthesia is administered to the skin and along the drainage tract, with a particular emphasis on anaesthetising the peritoneum. Using US guidance, an access needle is advanced into the collection. Two techniques can be applied to insert the drain tube – a direct 'stab' called the trocar technique or insertion of the tube over a guidewire using the Seldinger technique.
- For a large ascitic pocket or very well sonographically visualised intra-abdominal collection, the trocar technique can be safely used. US is used to guide the drainage catheter, which has a central sharp stylet, into the collection. Once in a satisfactory position, the sharp stylet and inner stiffener of the drainage catheter are removed allowing a pigtail to form (Fig. 15.3b). A drainage bag is then attached to the catheter and it is secured to the skin.
- The Seldinger technique, includes passage of a guidewire through an access needle. The needle is then exchanged over the guidewire for a drainage catheter (Fig. 15.1b) after first dilating the track to the abscess with fascial dilators.

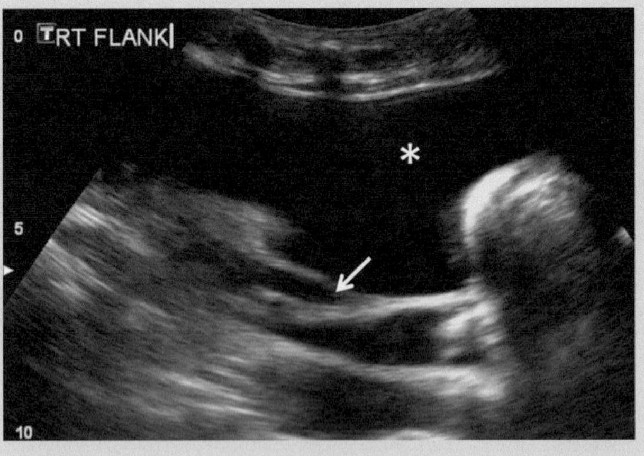

Fig. 15.2 Ultrasound of the right flank demonstrating a deep pocket of fluid (*asterisk*) with some loops of bowel visualised deep in the abdomen (*arrow*)

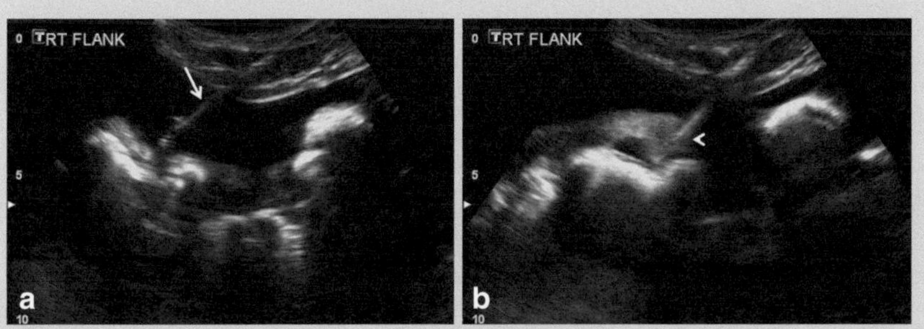

Fig. 15.3 (**a**) Abdominal ultrasound demonstrating a needle (*arrow*) being passed into the fluid collection under direct imaging guidance. (**b**) The drain is visualised coiled in the fluid collection (*arrow-head*)

Case 15.2

- A 40 year old male presented with right lower quadrant abdominal pain. The presence of a peri-appendiceal collection was confirmed on CT scan of the abdomen (Fig. 15.4). Due to its position and because of adjacent loops of bowel, CT guided drainage was performed. Again local anaesthesia is administered to the subcutaneous tissues and peritoneum. Then intermittent CT fluoroscopic images were obtained as the needle was advanced into the collection.

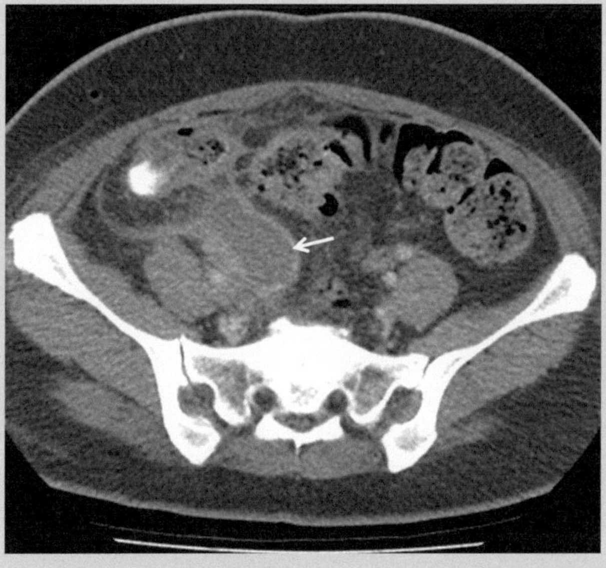

Fig. 15.4 CT of abdomen demonstrating an abscess (*arrow*) in the right hemipelvis secondary to perforated acute appendicitis

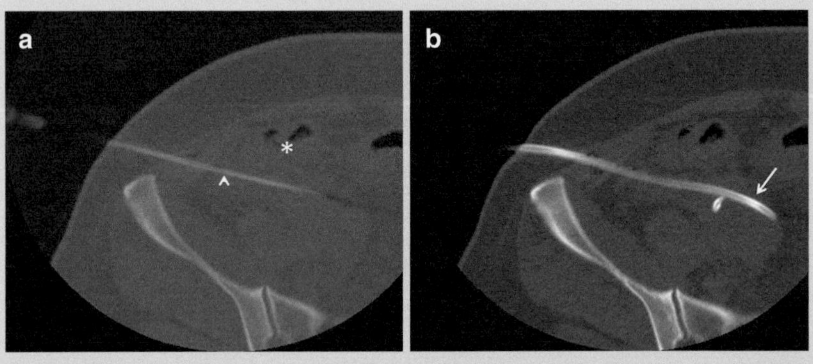

Fig. 15.5 (**a**) A needle (*arrow-head*) is advanced into the abscess under CT guidance using intermittent acquisitions. Note the safe access route behind the caecum (*asterisk*). (**b**) Final CT demonstrating the pigtail drain within the abscess (*arrow*)

- To confirm position, a sample was aspirated via the needle. Then the needle was exchanged over a guidewire and a drainage catheter inserted after dilating the track with fascial dilators. Tube position is confirmed by performing a final limited CT scan through the area (Fig. 15.5).

15.8 Post-procedure Care and Review

- Observation of vital signs and access site for local complications.
- Further treatment depends on the clinical condition of the patient. There is no indication for routine re-imaging of the patient if there is clinical improvement.
- If symptoms fail to resolve or recur post-procedure then repeat imaging is warranted:
- To assess the status of the collection
- To confirm the position of the drain.
- The calibre of the drain may need to be increased if there is particularly viscous contents.
- For viscous collections, intermittent irrigation can be used to ensure drain patency. It is performed by injection of 10–15 ml of sterile saline with an aseptic technique, followed by passive drainage or active aspiration. The exact volume is dependent on the site of drainage and the capacity of the potential space.
- If the drain blocks, it may require flushing with normal saline or fibrinolytics.
- Occasionally the drain may need to be re-sited due to migration of the drain, redistribution or change in the size and location of the collection pockets.
- The drain can be removed when drainage is less than 20 ml per day and if the patient is clinically well.

Key Points

- Imaged guided drainage is a minimally invasive and potentially life saving technique for accessing collections and can avoid the need for surgery in most cases.
- Ultrasound or CT imaging is used to select a safe access route to the collection and to guide catheter placement.
- By performing microbiological analysis on the sample, appropriate treatment regimens can be instigated.
- The drain should be monitored on a daily basis to ensure that it does not become blocked or displaced. Drain output should also be recorded on a daily basis.

Further Reading

1. Brown C, Kang L, Kim ST. Percutaneous drainage of abdominal and pelvic abscesses in children. Semin Intervent Radiol. 2012;29:286–94.
2. Frederick-Dyer K, Ahmad A, Arora, SS, Wile, G. Difficult biopsy and drainage: just say yes. Abdom Radiol (NY). 2016;41(4):706–19. doi:10.1007/s00261-016-0666-2.
3. Jaffe TA, Nelson RC. Image-guided percutaneous drainage: a review. Abdom Radiol (NY). 2016;41(4):629–36. doi:10.1007/s00261-016-0649-3.

16 Musculoskeletal Intervention

Damien O'Neill and Hamed Asadi

16.1 Introduction

- The musculoskeletal system comprises bones, joints, tendons, ligaments and their supporting neurovascular bundles. Disorders that affect the musculoskeletal system can be degenerative, infective, inflammatory, neoplastic or traumatic.
- A key component in evaluation of the musculoskeletal system is a detailed history and thorough examination, with subsequent radiological interventions for confirmation of diagnosis and treatment.
- MRI can provide exquisite details of the intra-articular and peri-articular structures. Certain joints e.g. the knee, usually have sufficient intrinsic contrast, making MRI assessment adequate. However sometimes for other joints, such as shoulder or hip, the administration of an intra-articular contrast agent to perform an MR arthrogram, can help in delineating the small structures of interest.

16.2 Joint Assessment

- The hip, knee and shoulder are the most common peripheral joints that are assessed radiologically. Initially plain radiograph assessment is usually performed. For evaluation of the intra-capsular structures, an arthrogram can be performed, and fluoroscopic guidance can be used to gain access to the joint.

D. O'Neill, MRCS, MMedSc (✉)
Department of Radiology, Beaumont Hospital, Dublin, Ireland
e-mail: damienconeill@rcsi.ie

H. Asadi, MD, PhD, FRANZCR, CCINR, EBIR
Interventional Neuroradiology Service, Austin Health, Melbourne, Victoria, Australia

School of Medicine, Faculty of Health, Deakin University, Victoria, Australia
e-mail: hamed.asadi@austin.org.au

H.K. Kok et al. (eds.), *Interventional Radiology for Medical Students*,
DOI 10.1007/978-3-319-53853-2_16

- If there is concern for joint infection, a sample of fluid should be aspirated and sent for microscopy and culture. A small amount of iodinated contrast material is then administered to confirm intra-capsular position.
- Therapeutic combinations of local anaesthetic and a corticosteroid can be administered, to treat joint inflammation or bursitis.
- For MR arthrograpy, a combination of 10–15 cc of normal saline and 0.1 cc Gadolinium based MRI contrast is instilled. The patient then undergoes an MR examination of the joint.

16.2.1 Indications for Joint Access

- Assessment of intra-articular structures, in particular, MR arthrogram.
- Diagnostic, therapeutic or palliative administration of medication.
- Therapeutic hydrostatic dilatation in adhesive capsulitis.
- Sampling of the joint contents.
- Therapeutic aspiration of the joint contents.
- Intracapsular irrigation.

16.2.2 Procedure Contraindications

There is no absolute contraindication and in case of suspected infective arthritis, sampling of the intracapsular content is inevitable. However the following should have further consideration:

- Infection over the access site or systemic sepsis.
- Recent fracture.
- Severe systemic coagulopathy (risk of haemarthrosis).
- Immunosuppression.
- Diabetes.

16.2.3 Patient Preparation

- Comprehensive review of symptoms, signs, investigations and imaging.
- Discussion with referring clinicians to ensure the correct procedure is performed and adequate samples are taken.
- Typically performed as an elective day case procedure.
- Blood investigations including a full blood count and coagulation studies.

16.2.4 Complications

- Infection
- Haemorrhage
- Chondrotoxicity (large doses of intra-articular steroids or certain anaesthetics)

Cases

- Fluoroscopic guided access of a shoulder joint prior to an MR arthrogram. The patient is positioned supine on a fluoroscopy Table. A sterile field is created. Local anaesthesia is administered to the skin and subcutaneous tissues.
- Using fluoroscopic guidance a 22 gauge spinal needle is advanced towards a bony landmark (usually 2/3 of the way down the humeral head, in its medial third) until contact is made with periosteum. At this stage, a sample can be aspirated or a small volume of iodinated contrast can be administered through the needle to confirm intra-articular position.
- A similar approach can be used for most synovial joints in the body.
- For aspiration of a suspected infected joint for diagnosis, the same technique is used to access the joint and a sample is aspirated and then sent for laboratory analysis.
- Similarly for therapeutic administration of intraarticular corticosteroids, a similar access technique is used and the mixture of analgesia is administered (Figs. 16.1, 16.2 and 16.3).

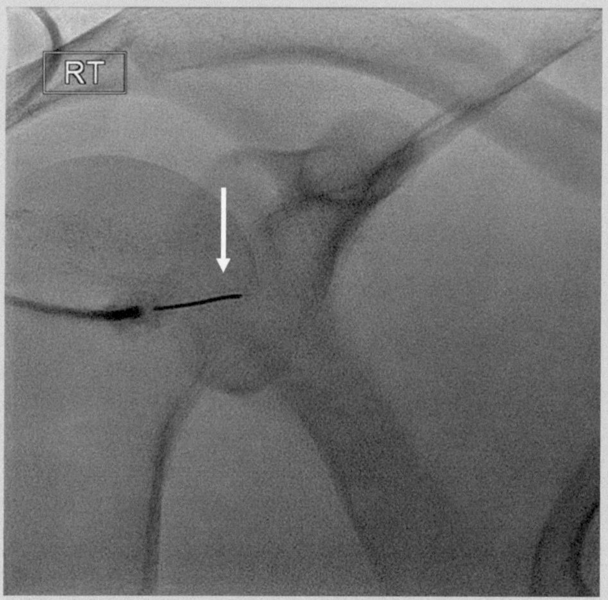

Fig. 16.1 Using fluoroscopy a 22 g spinal needle is advanced into the shoulder capsule, 2/3 of the way down the humeral head (*arrow*) until contact is made with periosteum

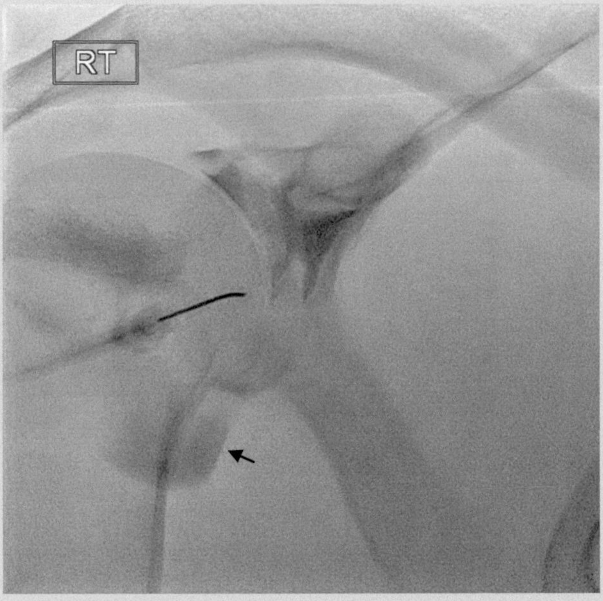

Fig. 16.2 A combination of iodinated contrast, local anaesthetic and gadolinium is injected. The iodinated contrast outlines the capsule of the joint confirming intra-articular position where contrast is seen to pool in the axillary recess (*arrow*)

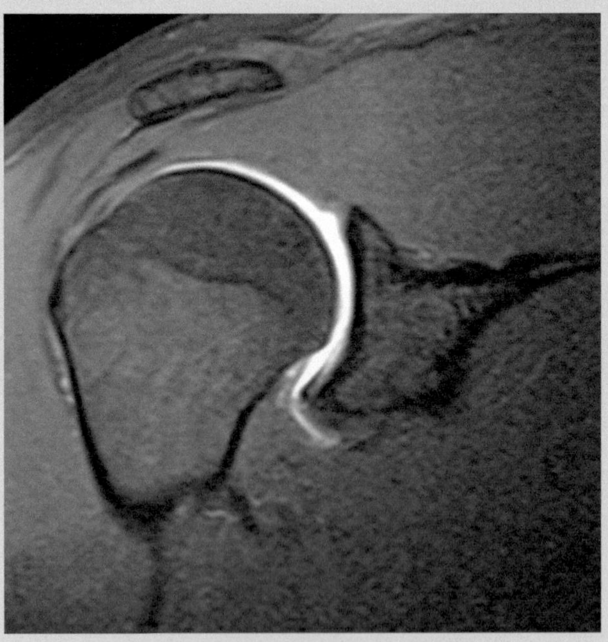

Fig. 16.3 Subsequent MR arthrogram with intra-articular gadolinium outlining the intra-articular structures. Axial and sagittal-oblique T1-fat saturated MRI sequences of the right shoulder

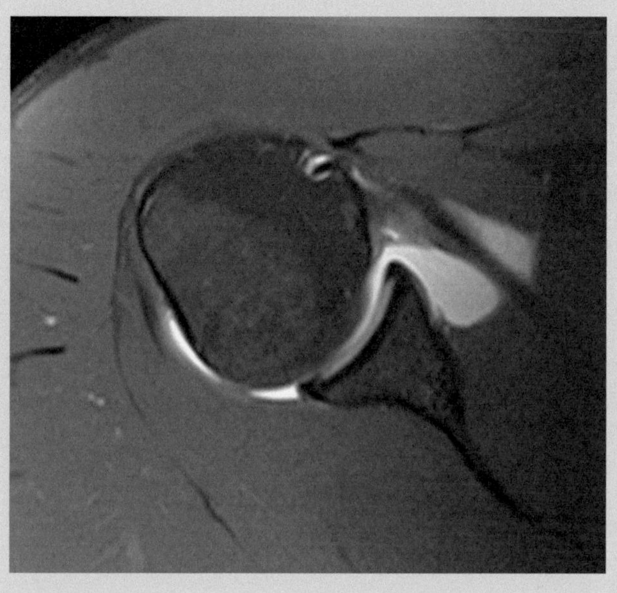

Fig. 16.3 (continued)

16.2.5 Post-procedure Care and Review

- Observation of vital signs and access site for local complications.
- Occasionally patients can get a local flare of pain and swelling which can last for a few hours post procedure.

16.3 Vertebroplasty

16.3.1 Introduction

- Osteoporotic fractures of the spine are often extremely painful and treatment comprises of immobilisation with a brace, analgesics and specific treatment of osteoporosis such as bisphosphonate therapy. However, further demineralisation can result from the immobilisation, thus accelerating the osteoporotic process at adjacent levels. Initial symptoms tend to resolve in 4–6 weeks, but some patients have severe, persistent pain for a long time.
- Later consequences of vertebral fractures are reduced height, kyphosis, and chronic back pain.
- Similarly, fractures from tumour metastases to the spine can be very painful, necessitating large analgesic requirements and the disease may progress with time. By treating these fractures, the analgesic requirement can be decreased in the frail elderly patient who is susceptible to the side-effects of opioid use.

- Vertebroplasty is a technique for treating a vertebral body fracture, typically as a result of osteoporosis or tumour. Under fluoroscopic guidance, bone cement e.g. poly-methyl-methacrylate (PMMA) is injected into the vertebral body. The theory behind this procedure is that the cement provides mechanical stabilisation at the fracture site and the heat emitted by the process of forming the cement destroys nearby nerve pain fibres aiding in analgesia.
- Kyphoplasty is a variation on vertebroplasty in which the lost height from a compression fracture is restored to the vertebra. Once access to the vertebra is achieved, balloons are inflated and then bone cement is injected into the space created to restore the height of the vertebra. Newer devices have also been recently introduced for this purpose, e.g. SpineJack.

16.3.2 Procedure Indications

- Osteoporotic fractures that have failed conservative management preferably within the acute phase (1–4 weeks of onset).
- Vertebral body invasion by tumour, usually metastatic.

16.3.3 Procedure Contraindications

- Asymptomatic fracture
- Active osteomyelitis of the target vertebra
- Un-correctable coagulopathy
- Allergy to vertebroplasty cement or contrast agent
- Significant central canal narrowing from retropulsion of bony fragments or epidural tumour.

16.3.4 Patient Preparation

- Comprehensive review of symptoms, signs, investigations and imaging.
- Discussion with the referring clinician; rheumatologist, geriatrician, oncologist, or surgeon.
- Typically performed as an elective inpatient procedure with best results occurring if performed within 10–14 days of the onset of pain.
- Performed under local anaesthesia and conscious sedation.
- Blood investigations including a full blood count and coagulation studies.
- Fasting from midnight before the day of intervention.
- Intravenous access, for IV sedation.

16.3.5 Complications

- Neurologic defect, from spinal canal or neural foraminal narrowing.
- Intravasation into the spinal venous plexus, IVC or even adjacent viscera.
- Pulmonary embolus form cement leakage into the systemic veins.
- Fracture of vertebral body, pedicles or rib.

- Infection.
- Allergic reaction.
- Haemorrhage.
- Pneumothorax or haemothorax.
- Spinal canal protrusion and cord damage.
- Hollow viscus or solid visceral injuries.

Case

- Vertebroplasty of a lower thoracic vertebra in an elderly patient with a wedge compression fracture secondary to osteoporosis, in whom conservative treatment had failed. A left transpedicular approach is used to access the vertebral body; position is confirmed on AP (Fig. 16.4a) and lateral (Fig. 16.4b) views.
- When a satisfactory position is obtained the bone cement (PMMA) is injected slowly into the vertebral body under fluoroscopic guidance. Injection is continued until the cement spreads evenly throughout the area of the vertebral body (Fig. 16.4c, d).
- Injection is normally ceased when sufficient cement has been administered or if cement is visualised outside the vertebral body e.g. vertebral venous plexus, spinal canal etc.

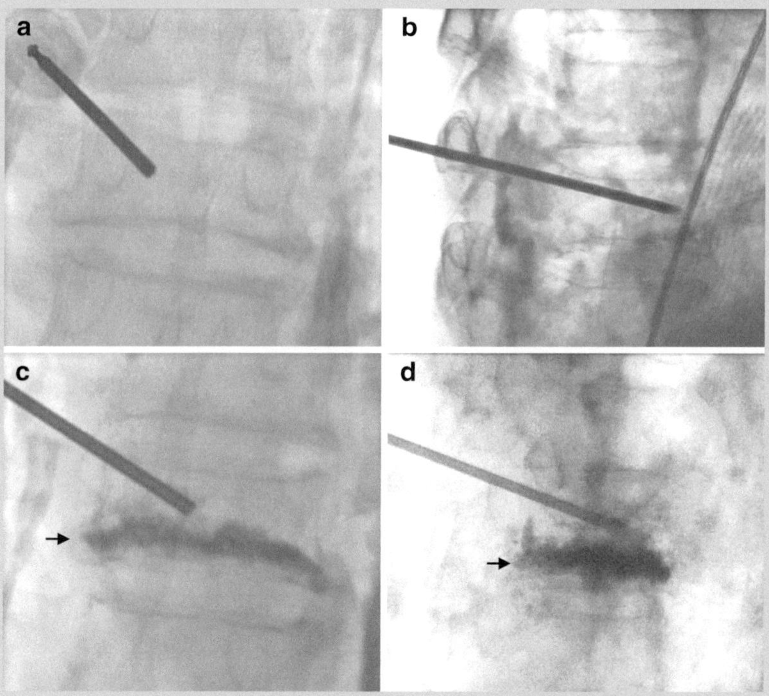

Fig. 16.4 (**a**) AP and (**b**) lateral views confirming position from a left transpedicular approach into the vertebral body. (**c**) AP and (**d**) lateral views demonstrating cement (*arrow*) after being injected into the vertebral body

Key Points

- Joint injections can be performed for diagnostic (e.g. aspiration of fluid, administration of contrast for arthrography) or therapeutic (e.g. therapeutic joint aspiration, administration of intraarticular corticosteroids) indications.
- MR arthrography involves the administration of dilute Gadolinium based contrast media into the joint under fluoroscopic guidance, followed by specific MR imaging sequences to allow evaluation of intra-articular structures.
- Vertebroplasty stabiles compression fractures of the vertebral column and provides analgesia to the patient.
- This is of benefit in an elderly population who are susceptible to the deleterious effects of prolonged opioid use, and detrimental effect of prolonged immobilisation. Multiple levels can be treated if needed.

16.3.6 Post-procedure Care and Review

- Observation of vital signs and access site for local complications.
- Monitor for any new neurological deficit or systemic complication.
- Frequently there may be additional vertebral levels that require treatment and this can be arranged after a short interval. Depending on patient tolerance and operator preference, multiple levels can be treated at one session.

16.3.7 Case Discussion

- Vertebroplasty is a minimally invasive procedure for the treatment of compression fractures of the vertebral bodies due to osteoporosis or metastatic invasion. Patients will have usually failed conservative treatment with analgesia and bracing.
- By performing a vertebroplasty, the need for other forms of analgesia (typically opiates) is reduced which is particularly beneficial in the elderly as they are more susceptible to adverse effects of opiate therapy.
- By injecting cement into the vertebral body, mechanical stability is increased and further loss of height can be prevented.
- A mechanism by which vertebroplasty is also postulated to have an effect is due to the thermal damage of adjacent pain sensory nerve fibres as the cement formation creates an exothermic reaction.
- If vertebral body height is to be restored, kyphoplasty can be performed.

Further Reading

1. Hansford BG, Stacy GS. Musculoskeletal aspiration procedures. Semin Intervent Radiol. 2012;29:270–85.
2. Stevenson M, et al. Percutaneous vertebroplasty and percutaneous balloon kyphoplasty for the treatment of osteoporotic vertebral fractures: a systematic review and cost-effectiveness analysis. Health Technol Assess. 2014;18:1–290.
3. Wang DT, Dubois M, Tutton SM. Complications in musculoskeletal intervention: important considerations. Semin Intervent Radiol. 2015;32:163–73.

Interventional Oncology

17

Elizabeth Ryan

17.1 Introduction

- Over the course of the last century, cancer treatment evolved to a complex multimodality care pathway delivered by a multidisciplinary team including radiology, surgical, medical oncology and radiation oncology specialists.
- There is a continuous drive towards cure or control of cancer via minimally invasive techniques, reducing patient morbidity and improving quality of life.
- Interventional Radiologists have developed endovascular and percutaneous techniques for locoregional cancer treatment.
- This has become known as the fourth pillar of cancer care.
- Interventional oncology (IO) is a rapidly evolving specialty with frequent development and innovation, both in terms of interventional techniques and in the scope of cancer treatment.
- Once thought limited to salvage therapy and palliation, ablative and embolisation therapy is approaching equivalence to standard first line surgical care for certain tumours.
- Given the significant difference in morbidity and hospital stay, it is expected that IO techniques may supersede surgery for appropriate tumours in time.
- Patient care encompasses pre-procedure consultation and decision-making, admission and treatment, and follow-up imaging and care.
- The interventional oncologist is a clinician familiar with the key facets of cancer care and is trained to diagnose and manage the side-effects and complications of their procedures.
- IO is broadly divided into endovascular therapy and percutaneous ablation.

E. Ryan
Department of Radiology, Beaumont Hospital and Royal College of Surgeons in Ireland, Dublin, Ireland
e-mail: lizryan1@gmail.com

H.K. Kok et al. (eds.), *Interventional Radiology for Medical Students*,
DOI 10.1007/978-3-319-53853-2_17

- Endovascular therapies involve access via the arterial system into the arteries suppling the tumour and direct delivery of chemotherapy and/or embolic material.
- Ablative techniques involve direct thermal or chemical destruction of the tumour via percutaneous delivery of an ablative device under image guidance.
- The principles of these techniques will be discussed, followed by examples of current clinical practice.

17.2 Percutaneous Ablative Image Guided Therapies in Cancer

- Image-guided tumour ablation involves placement of a wand-like probe into the tumour using image guidance and applying thermal or non-thermal energy to the tumour, resulting in cell death.
- Various modalities are in clinical practice and development of emerging therapies is ongoing.

17.2.1 Radiofrequency Ablation (RFA)

- A probe attached to a radiofrequency generator is inserted percutaneously directly into the tumour.
- An alternating current is delivering via the probe to the tumour tissue.
- Molecules constantly move to realign their poles with the alternating current.
- This motion produces friction, resulting in heating.
- Heating above 50 °C causes rapid permanent denaturation of cellular proteins and cell death via coagulative necrosis.
- The heat generated around the probe diminishes with distance, therefore the size of the ablation zone is limited.
- The ideal tumour size for one RFA probe is less than 3 cm, but the use of multiple probes can increase the ablation zone.
- Treatment efficacy may also be affected by heat loss into adjacent flowing blood. This is known as the heat-sink effect and occurs with very vascular tumours or tumours adjacent to large vessels.

17.2.2 Microwave Ablation

- Similar to RFA, an oscillating current is applied to a probe inserted into the tumour and the current induces molecular motion, friction and heating resulting in coagulative necrosis.
- Microwave ablation is less sensitive to the heat-sink effect than RFA and appears to be more protective of support tissues like the lining of the biliary tract and the renal collecting system and ureters.

17.2.3 Cryoablation

- Cryoablation is most commonly used in small renal malignancies and is also used in treatment of prostate cancer, soft tissue and bone tumours, liver and chest tumours.
- As for the other techniques, a probe is inserted percutaneously into the tumour.
- The technique involves rapid expansion of a gas flowing through and contained within the percutaneous probe which results in rapid cooling around the probe.
- Typically, two phases of cooling are separated by a phase of active thawing generated by a different gas flowing through the probe.
- This freeze-thaw-freeze cycle causes cell death by formation of extracellular and intracellular ice which disrupts membranes and causes protein denaturation, coagulation and vascular stasis, and apoptosis.

17.2.4 Irreversible Electroporation

- This is a new non-thermal ablative technique.
- Pulsed electric current is delivered to the tumour causing an increase in cellular membrane potential and resulting in the formation of multiple nanopores in the cell membrane.
- Irreversible disruption of the cell membrane results in cell death by a combination of apoptosis and coagulative necrosis.
- IRE causes muscular contraction and requires muscle relaxants to be administered by an anaesthetist. However, it is not associated with thermal injury or heat sink and it does not damage the extracellular support structures. It is also very fast, with a significantly shorter ablation time compared to the other techniques.

17.2.5 Chemical Ablation

- Percutaneous instillation of acetic acid or ethanol results in cell dehydration, protein denaturation and coagulative necrosis.
- Ethanol also causes destruction of vascular endothelium resulting in thrombosis and ischaemia.

17.2.6 Techniques for Protection of Surrounding Tissues

Ablative techniques, particularly thermal ablation, may result in injury to tissues adjacent to the ablation zone. There are several techniques to reduce the risk of injury.

Hydrodissection Fluid is injected between two structures to separate them, displacing important non-target structures away from the tumour intended for ablation. For example, a needle may be inserted

	into the fat between a renal tumour and the colon and injection of dextrose 5% fluid will displace the colon away from the tumour and provide a buffer for absorption of transmitted heat. CO_2 has also been used for this purpose.
Irrigation	Perfusion of cold fluid through a hollow structure adjacent to an ablation zone in order to keep the temperature at a safe level. For example, retrograde pyeloperfusion involves the placement of a ureteric stent into the renal pelvis and continuous irrigation with cold fluid while ablating a nearby renal tumour. This keeps the temperature within the renal pelvis and ureter below the level that would cause injury to these structures.

17.3 Endovascular Image Guided Therapies in Cancer

- The principle of transcatheter embolisation therapy is vascular occlusion to diminish or remove blood flow.
- There are myriad applications, from emergency embolisation for control of haemorrhage, to treatment of vascular malformations or varices, and tumour therapy.
- Within IO, transcatheter embolisation includes direct delivery of chemotherapy, occlusion of the suppling arteries to cause infarction of the tumour, and combination therapy with embolic material coated with chemotherapy or emitting radiation.

17.3.1 Embolic Agents

- There are a wide range of embolic material available categorised according to the level of occlusion desired and whether the effect should be temporary or permanent.
- Permanent agents are typically used in IO.

17.3.2 Temporary

17.3.2.1 Gelatin Sponge (Gelfoam)

- Water-insoluble porous sponge made from purified porcine skin gelatin.
- It is haemostatic and absorbable, the length of time to absorption depending onto the tissue into which is delivered (ranging from days to weeks).

17.3.3 Permanent

17.3.3.1 Particles

- These include polyvinyl alcohol particles (shavings of inert plastic) ranging from 50 to 2500 microns in size, and acrylic spheres ranging from 40 to 1300 microns.

17.3.3.2 Coils

- Stainless steel or platinum pieces of wire that are delivered through a catheter.
- These are manufactured to take a particular shape when released from the catheter and various coil shapes are available for different situations.

17.3.4 Transarterial Embolisation, Chemoembolisation and Radioembolisation

Options for tumour embolisation include:

- "Bland embolisation" / TransArterial Embolisation (TAE)
  - Embolisation without chemotherapy, resulting in tumour ischaemia and necrosis via occlusion of the blood supply.
- TransArterial ChemoEmbolisation (TACE)
  - Combination of delivery of chemotherapy and embolisation.
  - Local delivery allows high concentration drug delivery to the tumour with minimised systemic delivery and side effects.
  - Conventional TACE (cTACE) involves delivery of chemotherapy into the feeding arteries followed by embolisation with gelatin sponge or particles. The embolic agent helps to localise the chemotherapy in the tumour by reducing or eliminating blood flow, and also induces ischaemia and necrosis.
  - Drug-eluting bead TACE (DEB-TACE) involves delivery of particles containing with chemotherapy into the feeding arteries. These particles embolise the tumour, inducing ischaemia and necrosis, and slowly release the chemotherapy into the surrounding tissue over time.
- TransArterial RadioEmbolisation (TARE), also known as selective internal radiation therapy (SIRT)
  - Tumour embolisation with particles embedded with a beta-emitting radioactive isotope, yttrium-90 (Y-90). These radioactive beads emit short-range radiation locally into the tumour, allowing a significantly higher radiation dose than could be applied with external beam radiotherapy.

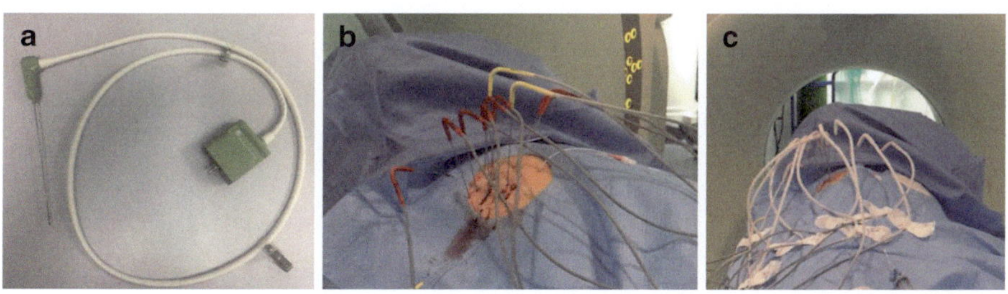

Percutaneous cryoablation. The patient is under general anaesthesia in the CT scanner. (**a**) Cryoprobe. (**b**) Multiple percutaneous cryoprobesin place. (**c**) Ice forming along the cryoprobe tubing

Interventional Oncology: Liver

18

Elizabeth Ryan

18.1 Hepatocellular Carcinoma (HCC)

- In patients with HCC the decision to opt for transplantation, surgical resection or ablation is multifactorial and complex, and each case is assessed on an individual basis at a multidisciplinary meeting (MDM).
- Factors that will aid decision making include tumour size, location, number of tumours, liver function, the predicted postoperative remaining liver volume and the patient's fitness for surgery.
- Ablation may offer cure in early-stage HCC but is limited by tumour size and location.
- Transarterial chemoembolisation (TACE) is considered for unresectable/unablatable HCC for the purpose of local control rather than cure. This may offer symptom improvement and lengthened survival. TACE may also be performed as a combination treatment to downsize a tumour and render it resectable or ablatable.
- Transarterial radioembolisation (also known as selective internal radiation therapy SIRT) is an emerging therapy also used for local control of incurable disease.

Early (A) stage Curative therapy (transplant/resection/ablation)

- Solitary tumour or up to 3 nodules <3 cm

Intermediate (B) stage Palliative therapy (TACE/TARE)

- Multinodular, unresectable, Child-Pugh A or B, performance status 0

E. Ryan
Department of Radiology, Beaumont Hospital and Royal College of Surgeons in Ireland, Dublin, Ireland
e-mail: lizryan1@gmail.com

H.K. Kok et al. (eds.), *Interventional Radiology for Medical Students*,
DOI 10.1007/978-3-319-53853-2_18

Advanced (C) stage Palliative therapy (Sorafenib)

- Portal vein invasion, nodal or distant metastases, performance status 1–2

18.2 Colorectal Cancer Liver Metastases (CRLM)

- Approximately 10–25% of patients with colorectal cancer are found to have liver metastases at the time of diagnosis, and a further 20–25% will subsequently develop liver metastases.
- Surgical resection may offer increased survival or even cure but only 25% of patients are suitable for resection.
- Historically, the remaining 75% were offered systemic chemotherapy to extend survival. More recently, various interventional oncology techniques have emerged which may offer increased survival and cure.
- Ablation is considered for patients with a limited number of hepatic metastases (ideally <4) of small size (<5 cm) who are unwilling or unsuitable to undergo surgical resection.
- As with HCC, transarterial therapies (TACE/TARE) are not considered curative in their own right, and have traditionally been used as salvage therapy when chemotherapy fails or to downstage metastases in order to permit surgical resection. Various chemotherapy combinations have been used, including doxorubicin, irinotecan, cisplatin, mitomycin C.
- Early studies of TARE in CRLM have shown efficacy in combination with systemic chemotherapy for salvage treatment after failure of first line chemotherapy.

18.3 GI Tract Neuroendocrine Tumours (NET)

- Gastroenteropancreatic neuroendocrine tumours are the second most prevalent GI tract neoplasm after colorectal cancer and most commonly occur in the small intestine, followed by the rectum, colon, pancreas, stomach and appendix.
- 60–80% have metastatic disease at presentation, most commonly to the liver.
- Interventional oncology techniques for NET liver metastases include ablation, TACE and TARE. Although data is limited, IO techniques are associated with improved survival.

18.4 Other Liver Metastatic Disease

- There is some data demonstrating safety and efficacy of locoregional therapies including ablation, TACE and TARE for liver metastases from melanoma, breast cancer, GI tumours and other malignancies but randomised controlled trials are necessary for a standardised approach.

18.5 IO Techniques for HCC and Liver Metastases

18.5.1 Ablation

18.5.1.1 Contraindications

- Diffuse/infiltrative tumours, vascular invasion, unresectable/unablatable extrahepatic metastatic disease.
- Uncorrectable coagulopathy.
- No safe percutaneous access route to the tumour(s) even with hydrodissection.
- Relative: proximity to gallbladder, stomach or bowel, or central location.

18.5.1.2 Patient Preparation

Imaging Contrast enhanced CT or MRI. Non-contrast, arterial and portal venous phases of the liver are required. CT should include chest and pelvis for staging.

MDM Multidisciplinary discussion including hepatology, hepatobiliary surgery, medical oncology and pathology. The patient's functional status and chronic liver disease should be factored into the treatment plan.

Lab Full blood count, coagulation status, liver biochemistry. International normalised ratio should be <1.5 and platelets $>50 \times 10^9$/L.

Medications If possible clopidogrel/warfarin/novel anticoagulant medications should be stopped 5 days prior.

Antibiotics If the patient has a colonised biliary tree (e.g. previous sphincterotomy/biliary stent/biliary-enteric anastomosis) there is an increased risk of abscess formation and periprocedural prophylactic antibiotic administration is recommended.

18.5.1.3 Technique

- RFA and microwave ablation are standard techniques for thermal ablation of HCC and liver metastases.
- Evidence suggests that there is less heat-sink with microwave ablation and a more predictable ablation zone and this is replacing RFA in many practices.
- There is a potential role for cryoablation, particularly for central/hilar tumours adjacent to bile ducts but there is less data.
- IRE is an emerging technique currently the subject of research in treatment of HCC.

18.5.1.4 Postprocedural Care

- Overnight hospital stay post-procedure is standard.
- A post-ablation syndrome including fever, nausea, vomiting and right upper quadrant pain is an expected side-effect of the procedure rather than a complication.
- Analgesia is administered as required.
- Routine follow-up imaging is performed to assess for recurrence.

Complications rate of 2–3%; mortality 0.1–0.5%.

- Subcapsular or intraperitoneal haemorrhage (0.5%)
- Hepatic abscess (0.3%)
- Bowel injury (0.2–0.3%)
- Haemothorax (<0.1%)
- Biloma (0.05–8%)
- Biliary injury – can result in stricture formation and chronic obstruction
- Thermal burns
- Iatrogenic cholecystitis related to proximity to ablation zone, usually self-limiting

18.5.2 TACE

18.5.2.1 Contraindications

- Advanced liver disease (Child-Pugh C, severe ascites, encephalopathy, active GI haemorrhage, hyperbilirubinaemia, hypoalbuminaemia, active hepatitis, poor performance status).
- Systemic issues including neutropaenia, cardiomyopathy and renal insufficiency.

18.5.2.2 Patient Preparation

- As for ablation.

18.5.2.3 Technique

- Treatment options include TAE, cTACE and DEB-TACE (see Introduction to Interventional Oncology) and there is no current consensus as to the best technique.
- Catheter inserted from the femoral artery into the common hepatic artery; angiograms performed to delineate tumoral arterial anatomy.
- A microcatheter is used to deliver selective treatment via small arterial branches supplying the tumour. Selective treatment in this manner minimises drug delivery to non-tumour liver tissue, an important factor in the setting of chronic liver disease.
- The particles are mixed with iodinated or oily contrast medium which can be visualised with fluoroscopy while injecting. The mixture is carefully injected until there is near stasis of flow.
- As previously described, haemostasis may be achieved at the common femoral artery access site with manual compression or with commercially available closure devices.

18.5.2.4 Postprocedural Care

- Regular measurement of vital statistics including heart rate and blood pressure for 4–6 h post-procedure. Overnight stay for observation and analgesia.
- The majority of patients experience some degree of postembolisation syndrome (nausea, abdominal pain and fever) which is related to a systemic inflammatory

response and tissue necrosis and requires only supportive treatment. Pain may last for up to a week.

- Antiemetics, analgesia and stool softeners.
- Routine follow-up imaging to assess for recurrence.

Complications rate 4–7% and mortality 1% in HCC; rate 30% and mortality 2% in CRLM.

- Access site – haemorrhage, pseudoaneurysm, arterial occlusion (<5%)
- Liver abscess (2–3%)
- Biloma (2%)
- Cholecystitis (5%)
- Non-target embolisation – GI tract embolisation results in ulcers which may be difficult to treat. (<5%)

18.5.3 Tare/SIRT

Patient preparation, interventional technique and postprocedural care are similar to TACE.

Complications as for TACE, with these additional considerations:

- Hepatotoxicity (15%)
- Significantly less postembolisation syndrome than is seen after TACE.
- Can be associated with radiation pneumonitis if there is shunting through the abnormal tumour vasculature to the lungs. (<1%)

Case

This patient has a new diagnosis of cirrhosis of the liver. A hepatocellular carcinoma was identified in the left lobe of the liver and the patient was not a candidate for transplantation.

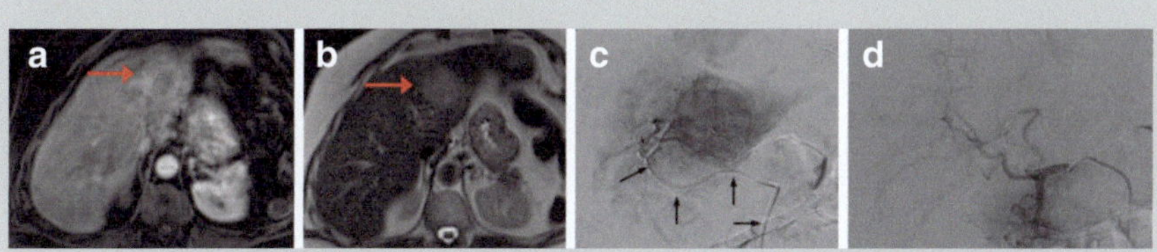

Transarterial chemoembolisation of hepatocellular carcinoma. (**a**, **b**) MRI with contrast shows an enhancing tumour in the liver (*arrows*). Enhancement in the arterial phase of imaging is typical of hepatocellular carcinoma. (**c**) An arterial catheter (*arrows*) has been passed from the common femoral artery (not seen) via the coeliac trunk, along the hepatic artery and into an artery supplying the tumour. Contrast injection shows tumour enhancement which is much greater than the surrounding liver. (**d**) With the catheter back in the common hepatic artery, contast injection shows that there is no longer evidence of tumour enhancement following successful embolisation

Key Points

- Hepatocellular carcinoma, colorectal and neuroendocrine liver metastases may be amenable to cure or palliation via ablation or transarterial treatments. Ablation may be curative, while transarterial techniques are usually palliative.
- There is some evidence for treatment of liver metastases from other primary tumours such as breast cancer and melanoma and research is ongoing.
- Treatment pathways are complex and evolve with new technologies, and all treatment should be planned via a multidisciplinary team approach using the best current evidence.

Suggested Reading

1. Clark T, Sabharwal T, editors. Interventional radiology techniques in ablation. Lee and Watkinson (Series Editors). London: Springer; 2013.
2. Kessel D, Ray CE, editors. Transcatheter embolisation and therapy. Lee and Watkinson (Series Editors). New York/London: Springer; 2010.
3. Kee ST, Murthy R, Madoff DC. Clinical interventional oncology. Philadelphia, PA: Elsevier; 2014.

Interventional Oncology: Renal Tumour Treatments

19

Elizabeth Ryan

- Surgery for primary malignant renal tumours has evolved from radical nephrectomy, through partial nephrectomy (PN) and laparoscopic nephrectomy.
- Tumours greater than 3 cm which take up intravenous contrast (i.e. "enhance") on CT or MRI are most likely malignant, usually renal cell carcinoma (RCC). However, enhancing masses <3 cm are benign in 25% of cases. Even for malignancies, at this small size the rate of growth and progression is slow.
- Management of small renal masses involves weighing the risk of life-altering disease progression against the morbidity of renal parenchymal loss associated with treatment, which is driving surgical management towards nephron-sparing surgery.
- IO techniques (primarily ablation) are associated with reduced morbidity, better preservation of renal volume and function, and improved recovery time.
- Emerging research suggests ablative techniques may have comparable oncologic outcomes with PN.
- While initially considered second line treatment for patients unfit for surgery, low morbidity and function preservation coupled with data suggesting oncologic equivalence confer an ever-increasing role in the management of small renal masses.

E. Ryan
Department of Radiology, Beaumont Hospital and Royal College of Surgeons in Ireland, Dublin, Ireland
e-mail: lizryan1@gmail.com

H.K. Kok et al. (eds.), *Interventional Radiology for Medical Students*,
DOI 10.1007/978-3-319-53853-2_19

19.1 Ablation

19.1.1 Current Indications

- Small renal mass <4 cm
- Increased risk of multiple RCCs (e.g. in von-Hippel-Lindau syndrome) where renal parenchymal preservation is vital
- Patient condition not suitable for surgery
- Solitary kidney

19.1.2 Patient Preparation

Clinical Thorough history and examination including risk factors for RCC, hereditary syndromes etc., prior surgery and general medical condition. The procedure should be discussed fully and informed patient consent given.

Labs Full blood count, renal function including eGFR, coagulation status. INR should be less than 1.5, platelet count should be greater than 50×10^9/L.

Imaging Contrast enhanced CT of the kidneys to evaluate the primary tumour and completion imaging of the remainder of the chest, abdomen and pelvis for metastatic disease.

NPO The patient should be fasting for at least 6 h pre-procedure.

19.1.3 Contraindications

- Uncorrectable coagulopathy.
- Metastatic disease – this is a relative C/I as there is an emerging role for ablation of certain metastases.
- No safe route to the tumour even with techniques like hydrodissection.

19.1.4 Technique

- Radiofrequency (RFA), microwave (MWA) and cryoablation are all acceptable techniques for percutaneous ablation of renal tumours.
- Advantages of MWA include faster ablation and larger, more homogenous ablation zones than RFA.
- Cryoablation appears to be relatively protective of the support structures including hilar vasculature and the collecting system.
- The choice of technique is largely down to the experience of the operator and availability of equipment.
- Technique is as described previously (see Introduction to Interventional Oncology).

- Hydrodissection has an important role particularly for tumours in proximity to the colon in the anterior kidney.
- Pyeloperfusion is helpful for thermal techniques used adjacent to the renal collecting system to prevent injury and long term complications such as ureteric strictures.

19.1.5 Postprocedural Care

- Overnight hospital stay post-procedure is standard.
- Analgesia is administered as required.
- Routine follow-up imaging is performed to assess for recurrence.

19.1.6 Complications

Minor Pain, paraesthesia, transient haematuria, transient chyluria and subcapsular haematoma. (all 1–5%)

Major Haemorrhage requiring transfusion and/or embolisation (1% for RFA and MWA, 5% for cryoablation), collecting system or ureter injury (1.5%), abscess and bowel injury (both <1%), pneumothorax (2%).

19.2 Embolisation

- Embolisation is mainly indicated as part of a combined approach with surgical or ablative techniques in order to downsize a renal cell cancer tumour or as palliation for intractable haematuria in patients with inoperable tumours.
- Renal cell carcinomas are typically very vascular tumours and preoperative embolisation may render surgical resection safer.
- Pre-ablation embolisation may reduce the heat-sink effect found with RFA and render this technique more effective.

19.2.1 Technique

- Similar to liver embolisation, selective angiography of the renal arteries is followed by superselective catheterisation of the branches feeding the tumour.
- The choice of embolic agent is influenced by the characteristics of the tumour and the vascularity of the kidney. Agents include ethanol or embolic particles.
- Pre-procedure workup and post-procedure care are similar to the previously described transarterial therapies. As with liver embolisation, most patients will experience some degree of post-embolisation syndrome which is self-limiting with supportive care.

Case

A 76 year-old patient had an incidental finding of a small renal tumour on CT. Surveillance imaging showed interval tumour growth, therefore treatment was indicated. However, the patient was not fit for surgical resection due to multiple medical co-morbidities and percutaneous microwave ablation was performed, with a good outcome.

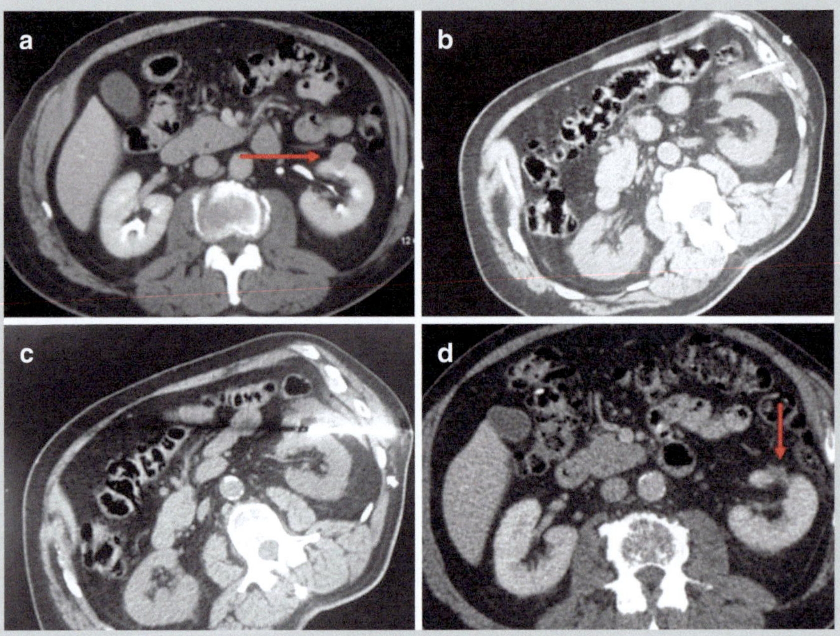

Percutaneous renal tumour microwave ablation. (**a**) Post-contrast CT demonstrates a partially exophytic mass at the anterior interpolar region of the left kidney (*arrow*). There are loops of bowel anterior to the tumour. (**b**) A needle has been introduced into the fat between the renal tumour and the nearby bowel loops and dextrose injected to separate them. This is known as hydrodissection. (**c**) A microwave probe has been inserted into the tumour for ablation. (**d**) Follow-up post-contrast CT shows the tumour is no longer seen and there is a focal scar at the site (*arrow*)

Key Points

- Small renal tumours are usually quite indolent and 1 in 4 are benign, therefore nephron-sparing low-morbidity treatments are preferable.
- IO techniques (primarily ablation) are associated with reduced morbidity, better preservation of renal volume and function, and improved recovery time.
- Currently percutaneous ablation is considered for patients unfit for surgery or with single kidneys or a predisposition to multiple renal tumours. Partial nephrectomy remains first-line treatment for patients fit for surgery but this treatment algorithm is in evolution as emerging evidence suggests that ablation therapies have similar outcomes to surgery.
- Ablation techniques include RFA, MWA and cryoablation.
- Embolisation is not curative for renal tumours and is typically used for devascularisation prior to surgery or ablation, to treat acute haemorrhage or palliate symptoms of intractable haematuria.

Suggested Reading

1. Chang X, et al. Radiofrequency ablation versus partial nephrectomy for clinical T1b renal cell carcinoma: long-term clinical and oncologic outcomes. J Urol. 2015;193(2):430–5.
2. Clark T, Sabharwal T, editors. Interventional radiology techniques in ablation. Lee and Watkinson (Series Editors). New York/London: Springer; 2013.
3. Kee ST, Murthy R, Madoff DC. Clinical interventional oncology. Philadelphia, PA: Elsevier; 2014.
4. Kessel D, Ray CE, editors. Transcatheter embolisation and therapy. Lee and Watkinson (Series Editors). Springer; 2010.

20 Interventional Oncology: Other

Elizabeth Ryan

20.1 Thoracic Interventional Oncology

- Surgical resection is the first line therapy for treating primary and metastatic pulmonary malignancy with curative intent.
- Percutaneous ablation is an alternative treatment offering a survival advantage in non-surgical candidates, with benefits over surgery including better preservation of normal lung parenchyma and lower treatment-related morbidity. Furthermore it is not necessary to suspend chemotherapy to undergo ablation.

20.1.1 Indications

- **Primary-**early stage disease (stage I and II disease; International Association for the Study of Lung Cancer IASLC 7th edition).
- **Metastases-**up to 5 less than 5 cm each, ideally less than 3.5 cm.
- **Medical comorbidities-**non-operative candidates.

20.1.2 Technical Considerations

Tumours results are best for tumours surrounded by normal lung. Tumours abutting the pleura can be treated but this will cause increased periprocedural pain.

Heat sink results are less successful for tumours adjacent to vessels of 3 mm diameter or greater.

E. Ryan
Department of Radiology, Beaumont Hospital and Royal College of Surgeons in Ireland, Dublin, Ireland
e-mail: lizryan1@gmail.com

H.K. Kok et al. (eds.), *Interventional Radiology for Medical Students*,
DOI 10.1007/978-3-319-53853-2_20

Air aerated lungs has an insulating effect. This results in better heating in the centre of the ablation zone but limits ablation at the periphery, which must be taken into account when planning the ablation zone margin.

Route As for lung biopsy, a route to the tumour should be carefully planned that will be technically feasible without crossing fissures (this increases the risk of pneumothorax), or major vascular structures.

20.1.3 Patient Preparation

Clinical Thorough history and examination including indicators of pulmonary function, prior surgery and general medical condition. Many of these patients are smokers with associated cardiovascular comorbidities. The procedure should be discussed fully and informed patient consent given.

Labs Full blood count, coagulation status. INR should be less than 1.5, platelet count should be greater than 70×10^9/L.

Imaging Contrast-enhanced CT of the chest to evaluate the primary tumour and completion imaging of the abdomen and pelvis for metastatic disease.

NPO The patient should be fasting for 6 h pre-procedure.

20.1.4 Contraindications

- Uncorrectable coagulopathy.
- No safe route to the tumour.
- Poor respiratory function or severe bullous emphysema rendering the procedure unsafe with the patient being unable to tolerate a post-procedure pneumothorax.
- Other untreatable metastatic disease.

20.1.5 Technique

- RFA is the most established technique for percutaneous ablation in the chest but MWA and cryoablation have been proved safe and efficacious and the choice of technique is largely down to operator experience and preference.

20.1.6 Postprocedure Care

- The patient should lie supine or procedure-side-down for 4 h following the procedure to reduce the risk of pneumothorax.
- Pain relief is administered as required for less painful procedures; whereas patient-controlled opioid analgesia may be of benefit for pleural and chest wall

ablations. Otherwise postprocedure care is as described previously for abdominal ablation.

- A mild postablation syndrome characterised by low-grade fever and malaise is common and self-limiting.

20.1.7 Complications

- Pneumothorax is common (11–50%), chest drain required for 6–25%, bronchopleural fistula in 0.6%
- Pleural effusion (6–20%)
- Haemoptysis (3–9%), all intrathoracic haemorrhage including haemothorax 5–20%
- Thermal injury to the chest wall, recurrent laryngeal, phrenic, intercostal and brachial plexus nerves and skin (0.5–1.5%)
- Air embolism (<1%)

20.2 Prostate Cancer

- Prostate cancer is a common cancer ranging from low-grade low-volume incidental disease to high-grade progressive disease with considerable mortality.
- The goal of prostate cancer care is to identify those cancers that require treatment, and to treat with intent to cure while minimising morbidity.
- Prostate cancer is often multifocal and focal treatments aim to target the index or dominant lesion as it is taken to represent the most aggressive focus of disease.
- Focal treatments include image-guided cryoablation and other new techniques under development including high-intensity focused ultrasound (HIFU), photodynamic therapy, laser ablation.

20.3 Ovarian Cancer

- There is a survival benefit with tumour debulking, or "cytoreduction" even in advanced stage ovarian cancer.
- As with surgical debulking, IO techniques cannot currently offer a cure for advanced disease but may improve survival via cytoreduction. Very limited studies suggest the safety and efficacy of ablative techniques like RFA, MWA and cryoablation for local control and palliation.

20.4 Benign Bone Lesions

- Many benign bone lesions are readily diagnosed on imaging, predominantly plain radiographs, and the majority are incidental asymptomatic findings which do not require management.

- For a small number of patients, benign bone lesions may result in pain or pathological fractures.
- Percutaneous ablation offers relief of symptoms with the morbidity and recovery associated with surgery. For example, percutaneous ablation is now a curative first-line treatment for osteoid osteomas, a benign bone lesion which presents with pain.

20.5 Musculoskeletal Malignancy

- Indications for percutaneous ablation in bone malignancy include pain relief, halting local progression into critical structures and stabilisation of collapsing pathological vertebral fractures.
- Previously described ablation techniques may be used for primary and secondary bone tumours, as well as cementoplasty which has benefits for structural support and pain relief. This involves injection of bone cement directly into the tumour via an image-guided percutaneous needle (See chapter on Musculoskeletal intervention).

Suggested Reading

1. Clark T, Sabharwal T, editors. Interventional radiology techniques in ablation. Lee and Watkinson (Series Editors). Philadelphia, PA: Springer; 2013.
2. Kee ST, Murthy R, Madoff DC. Clinical interventional oncology. Philadelphia, PA: Elsevier; 2014.
3. Kessel D, Ray CE, editors. Transcatheter embolisation and therapy. Lee and Watkinson (Series Editors). New York/London: Springer; 2010.

Carotid Angioplasty and Stenting (CAS) 21

Hamed Asadi

21.1 Introduction

- Ten percent of acute ischemic strokes (AIS) are due to severe carotid artery stenosis, making carotid revascularization one of the most important therapeutic managements in ischemic stroke.
- Older guidelines had reserved carotid artery stenting (CAS) for severe stenosis in symptomatic patients considered high risk for carotid endarterectomy (CEA).
- These guidelines were based on multiple previous trials including the North American Symptomatic Carotid Endarterectomy Trial (NASCET) and European Carotid Surgery Trial (ECST) that provided evidence of the superiority of CEA as the best medical therapy for symptomatic patients.
- However, the recent long-term results from the Carotid Revascularization Endarterectomy Versus Stenting Trial (CREST), with over 10-years comprehensive follow-up, did not find a significant difference between patients who underwent stenting versus those who underwent endarterectomy with respect to the risk of peri-procedural stroke, myocardial infarction, or death, as well as subsequent ipsilateral stroke. Also, the rate of post-procedural ipsilateral stroke also did not differ between the two groups.
- This equipoise likely benefitted from increasing refinement in CAS device technology and improving techniques over the past decade.
- The jury is still out for asymptomatic patients, as the current evidence for this group of patients, based on Asymptomatic Carotid Atherosclerosis Study (ACAS) and the Asymptomatic Carotid Surgery Trial (ACST), is of CEA superiority in patients with more than 60% carotid stenosis, with approximately 5.5% reduction in 5-year stroke risk over CAS.

H. Asadi, MD, PhD, FRANZCR, CCINR, EBIR
Interventional Neuroradiology Service, Austin Health, Melbourne, Victoria, Australia

School of Medicine, Faculty of Health, Deakin University, Victoria, Australia
e-mail: hamed.asadi@austin.org.au

H.K. Kok et al. (eds.), *Interventional Radiology for Medical Students*,
DOI 10.1007/978-3-319-53853-2_21

- The most important question about patients with asymptomatic significant carotid stenosis, recently defined as more than 70%, is whether medical treatment alone is sufficient or inferior to combined medical therapy and surgical intervention, and if inferior whether there is equipoise between CAS and CEA.
- This is the question that the CREST-2 study is trying to answer by 2020.

21.1.1 Procedural Risk and Risk Reduction Strategies

- In addition to operator experience, procedural volumes have a direct impact on the outcome of CAS.
- There are different factors influencing the overall risk associated with carotid artery stenting including anatomic features such as echo-lucent plaques, unfavourable aortic arches, tortuous vessels, lesion calcification, and complex lesions, as well as procedural time which may prolong catheter and guidewire manipulation within a fragile vascular bed.
- Embolisation protection devices (small removable filters placed during stent placement) have been proven to be beneficial in prevention of peri-procedural distal thromboembolic events, by making retrieval of iatrogenic debris possible with an astonishing relative risk reduction of greater than 50%.
- There are individual differences in peri-procedural medication for CAS depending on the local hospital policy and guideline. However, patients should usually be medicated at least 1 day prior to intervention with combined Asprin (75–600 mg) and Clopidogrel (300–600 mg); followed by on the Table IV infusion of 80 IU/kg heparin (5000–7000 IU) just before the guide wire is advanced into the carotid artery.
- Depending on local policies and guidelines, post-procedurally patients are prescribed daily Clopidogrel (75 mg) and Aspirin (75–150 mg) for at least 30 days (usually 6–12 months) followed by daily Aspirin only indefinitely.

21.2 Procedure Indications

There is no definite consensus on the indications for carotid artery stenting; however, following recent trials showing non-inferiority of CAS compared with CEA, the indications are rapidly growing:

- Crescendo TIAs with significant carotid stenosis.
- Intermittent TIAs due to significant carotid stenosis, non-responsive to medical management.
- Acute stroke for thrombectomy with or without tandem occlusion, with underlying severe carotid stenosis.
- Flow limiting or symptomatic carotid dissection.
- Traumatic carotid injuries with pseudoaneurysm, which usually require a covered stent.

- Cerebral hypo-perfusion with intermittent neurological symptoms due to severe underlying carotid stenosis. Although still under investigation, there is emerging evidence for the potential role of cerebral hypo-perfusion in causing cognitive decline due to severe carotid stenosis.
- Established infarction with underlying carotid stenosis maybe subjected to stenting depending on the extent of the abnormalities, and usually in a delayed fashion.

21.3 Procedure Contraindications

- Lack of expertise or unavailability of the required technology.
- Recent large established infarction at the time of presentation.
- Complete arterial occlusion.
- Contraindication for proper antiplatelet treatment.
- Impossible access or cannulation.

21.4 Patient Preparation

- Dynamic carotid stenosis interrogation by US, with Doppler velocity assessment.
- Patient should preferably have cross sectional angiographic imaging, preferably a CT angiogram from the aortic arch to the vertex of the skull.
- Routine blood tests, including coagulation profile.
- Dual antiplatelet therapy prior to the procedure, depending on institutional protocols.
- Platelet sensitivity-reactivity assessment just before the procedure, depending on the institutional availability

21.5 Complications

The overall complication risk is usually considered less than 6% if the procedure is performed in an experienced institution:

- Thromboembolism and resultant ischemic stroke.
- Vasovagal and asystole.
- Carotid dissection, tear or occlusion.
- Stent malposition.
- Stent fracture or occlusion.
- Chronic stent induced thromboembolism.
- In-stent stenosis.
- Groin complications.
- Reperfusion syndrome and intrarenal haemorrhage.
- Complications secondary to pre- or post- operative antiplatelet or anticoagulation treatment.
- Death.

21.6 Case Study

- Seventy-five-year-old male patient presented with crescendo TIAs with a right sided hemiparesis. He was diagnosed with multilevel high grade left internal carotid artery stenoses, confirmed on US, with no evidence of a visible acute infarction or haemorrhage on his CT brain. He received 600 mg of Asprin and 600 mg of Clopidogrel 4 days prior to the procedure (Fig. 21.1).
- This patient had 2 stenoses on angiography and 2 stents were placed after first inserting a filter to trap any debris dislodged during the procedure
- Gentle remodelling at the level of the inserted stents was performed using a 5 mm balloon. This is because when stents are deployed through a narrowed area, they conform to the internal dimensions of the lumen. Therefore, the stent will have a waist in the area of the stenosis which requires balloon expansion.
- In some centres during balloon expansion of the stent, the patient is asked to squeeze a squeaky rubber duck in his contralateral hand intermittently to ensure his level of consciousness and intact motor function.
- Final angiographic runs demonstrated a good radiographic result (Figs. 21.1 and 21.2) with no complications and normal intracranial arteries. Patient remained on dual antiplatelet therapy for 6 months, followed by 75 mg aspirin daily for life.

21.7 Post-procedure Care and Review

- Post-operatively patients are usually transferred to specialised neurology wards; however, depending on the clinical status and potential procedural complications high dependency or neurointensive care may be required for close monitoring of clinical status and vital parameters, e.g. BP.
- All immediate postop patients require regular monitoring of the arterial puncture site and limb vascular assessment, as per protocol.
- All postop patients require regular neurological assessment, as per institutional protocol.
- Dual antiplatelet therapy should be continued, depending on the institutional experience and protocol for 3–6 months, usually followed by 75 mg of Aspirin only for life.
- Patients with crescendo TIAs, usually remain as inpatients for at least 2 days, then depending on their recovery post stenting, can be discharged home.
- There is no universal consensus regarding postop followup, but repeat CT or CT angiogram is generally not recommended in immediate post-op period unless there is clinical concern.
- Depending on institutional protocols, long term follow-up imaging can be performed by annual Duplex US to assess for potential restenosis or in-stent complications.

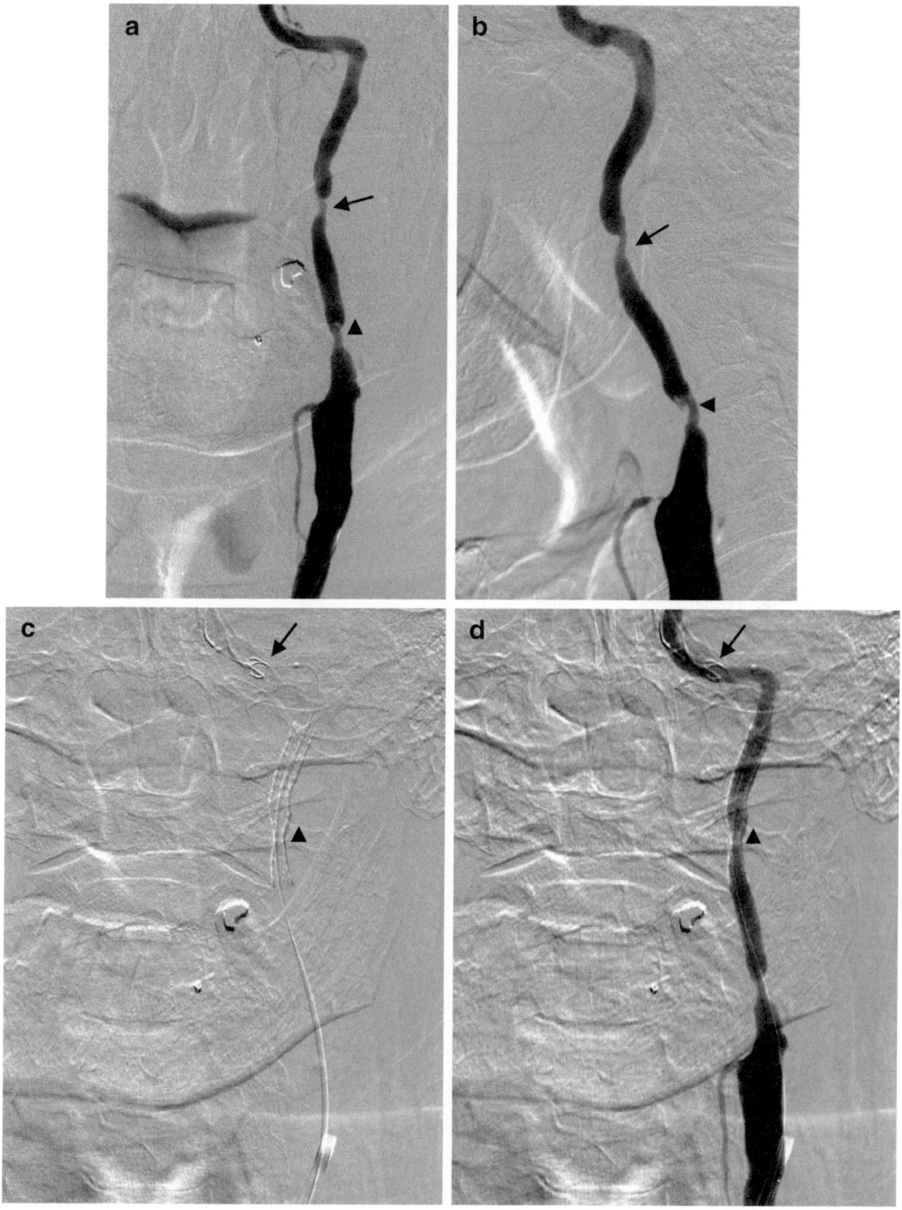

Fig. 21.1 Left CCA frontal (**a**) and lateral (**b**) angiograms demonstrating near complete ECA occlusion and severe proximal (*Arrowhead*) and distal (*Arrow*) cervical ICA stenoses. (**c**, **d**) demonstrating filter-wire at the base of the skull (*Arrow*) with stenting of the distal stenosis (*Arrowhead*); followed by further proximal stent insertion (*Arrowhead*) on (**e**, **f**)

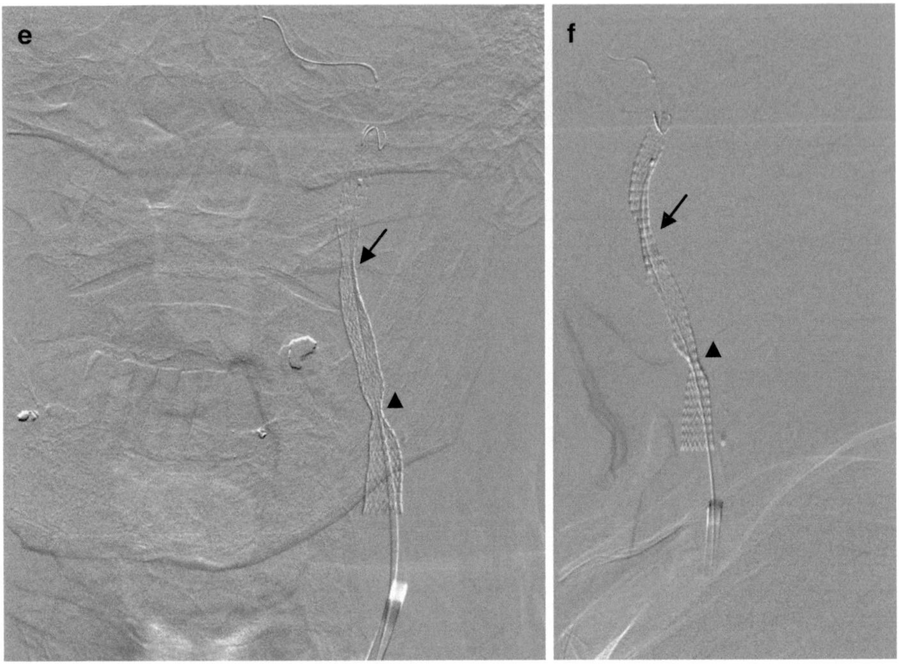

Fig. 21.1 (continued)

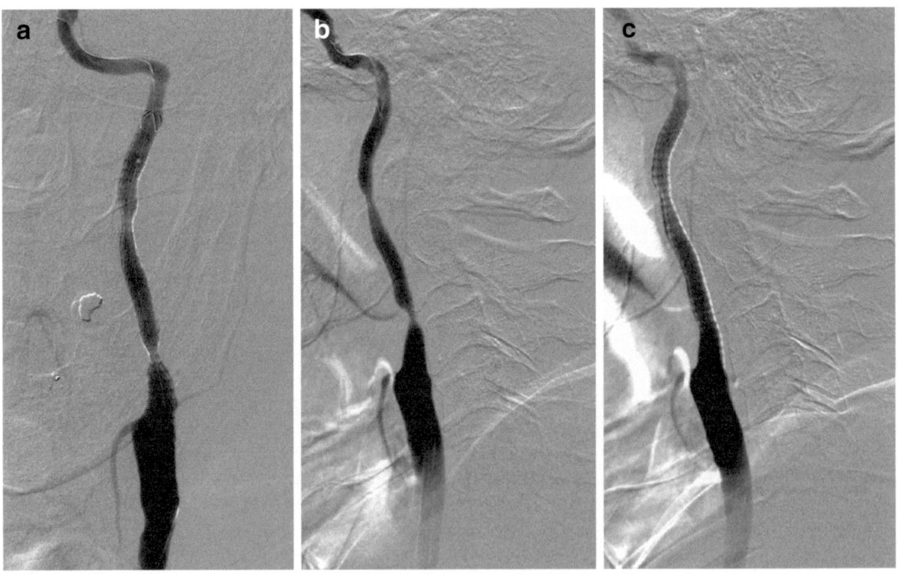

Fig. 21.2 Very good positioning of the both stent shown on AP and Lateral injections (**a**, **b**), with residual narrowing which responded well to the subsequent balloon remodelling (**c**) with excellent final angiographic result

21.8 Case Discussion

- Transient Ischemic Attack (TIA) is a relatively common medical condition; however, the exact definition of the condition is a matter of controversy with a new school of thought emerging debating its existence as an entity distinct from the ischemic stroke syndrome.
- Parallel to overall increasing prevalence of atherosclerotic diseases, there is an undeniable increase in the incidence of carotid stenosis, which is potentially one of the sources of thromboembolism in TIA and acute ischemic stroke (AIS) as well as in patients with chronic cerebral hypo-perfusion.
- Given the potential risk of AIS and its high mortality and morbidity, intervention is imperative in severe carotid stenosis.
- Severity of the carotid stenosis depends on its potential haemodynamic effect. This can be assessed using CT or MR angiographic techniques which can investigate the luminal narrowing or presence of atherosclerotic plaques, or alternatively can be evaluated with doppler US by measuring the blood flow velocity.
- Although not universally accepted, filter-wires have been shown to have a protective effect against distal thromboembolism during carotid stent placement.
- Any endoluminal manipulation around the carotid bifurcation or ICA bulb can result in a vasovagal response and profound bradycardia, which may require pharmacological reversal, i.e. Atropine (300–600 μg), which should be on hand.
- Patient should continue dual antiplatelet therapy for a period of 3–6 month followed by Asprin for life.

Key Points

- Acute stroke is a relatively common clinical condition with potential catastrophic outcome, which sometimes can present with prodromal episodes of TIAs.
- One of the common causes of TIAs is atherosclerotic stenosis of the ICA.
- CAS has been through a tempestuous research journey and is sometimes thought to be the most comprehensively studied and skeptically interrogated medical technique in the history of medicine
- However, the most recent CREST results have demonstrated an overall unequivocal equipoise between CAS and CAE, which is most likely going to maximise the role of CAS.
- Premedication and post-op antiplatelet therapy is essential for patients with planned CAS.

Suggested Reading

1. Barnett HJ, Taylor DW, Eliasziw M, Fox AJ, Ferguson GG, Haynes RB, et al. Benefit of carotid endarterectomy in patients with symptomatic moderate or severe stenosis. N Engl J Med. 1998;339(20):1415–25.
2. Brott TG, Halperin JL, Abbara S, Bacharach JM, Barr JD, Bush RL, et al. 2011 ASA/ACCF/AHA/AANN/AANS/ACR/ASNR/CNS/SAIP/SCAI/SIR/SNIS/SVM/SVS guideline on the management of patients with extracranial carotid and vertebral artery disease: a report of the American College of Cardiology Foundation/American Heart Association task force on practice guidelines, and the American Stroke Association, American Association of Neuroscience Nurses, American Association of Neurological Surgeons, American College of Radiology, American Society of Neuroradiology, Congress of Neurological Surgeons, Society of Atherosclerosis Imaging and Prevention, Society for Cardiovascular Angiography and Interventions, Society of Interventional Radiology, Society of NeuroInterventional Surgery, Society for Vascular Medicine, and Society for Vascular Surgery Developed in collaboration with the American Academy of Neurology and Society of Cardiovascular Computed Tomography. J Am Coll Cardiol. 2011;57(8):e16–94.
3. Brott TG, Howard G, Roubin GS, Meschia JF, Mackey A, Brooks W, et al. Long-term results of stenting versus endarterectomy for carotid-artery stenosis. N Engl J Med. 2016;374(11):1021–31.
4. Collaborators NASCET. Beneficial effect of carotid endarterectomy in symptomatic patients with high-grade carotid stenosis. N Engl J Med. 1991;325(7):445–53.
5. Enomoto Y, Yoshimura S. Antiplatelet therapy for carotid artery stenting. Interve Neurol. 2013;1(3–4):151–63.
6. Garg N, Karagiorgos N, Pisimisis GT, Sohal DP, Longo GM, Johanning JM, et al. Cerebral protection devices reduce periprocedural strokes during carotid angioplasty and stenting: a systematic review of the current literature. J Endovasc Ther. 2009;16(4):412–27.
7. Group MACSTC. Prevention of disabling and fatal strokes by successful carotid endarterectomy in patients without recent neurological symptoms: randomised controlled trial. Lancet. 2004;363(9420):1491–502.
8. Hobson RW, Howard VJ, Brott TG, Howard G, Roubin GS, Ferguson R. Organizing the carotid revascularization endarterectomy versus stenting trial (crest): national institutes of health, health care financing administration, and industry funding. Curr Control Trials Cardiovasc Med. 2001;2(4):160–4.
9. Hopkins LN, Roubin GS, Chakhtoura EY, Gray WA, Ferguson RD, Katzen BT, et al. The carotid revascularization endarterectomy versus stenting trial: credentialing of interventionalists and final results of lead-in phase. J Stroke Cerebrovasc Dis. 2010;19(2):153–62.
10. Investigators A. Endarterectomy for asymptomatic carotid artery stenosis. Executive Committee for the Asymptomatic Carotid Atherosclerosis Study. JAMA. 1995;273(18):1421–8.
11. Lal B, Meschia J, Brott T. CREST-2: guiding treatments for asymptomatic carotid disease. Endovascular Today. 2013:73–6.
12. Lam RC, Lin SC, DeRubertis B, Hynecek R, Kent KC, Faries PL. The impact of increasing age on anatomic factors affecting carotid angioplasty and stenting. J Vasc Surg. 2007;45(5):875–80.
13. Lloyd-Jones D, Adams RJ, Brown TM, Carnethon M, Dai S, De Simone G, et al. Heart disease and stroke statistics—2010 update a report from the American Heart Association. Circulation. 2010;121(7):e46–e215.
14. Macdonald S, Lee R, Williams R, Stansby G. Towards safer carotid artery stenting a scoring system for anatomic suitability. Stroke. 2009;40(5):1698–703.
15. Vogel TR, Dombrovskiy V. Carotid artery stenting in the nation: the influence of hospital and physician volume on outcomes. Vasc Endovasc Surg. 2009;45(2):205.

22 Acute Ischemic Stroke

Hamed Asadi

22.1 Introduction

- Stroke is considered one of the major public health problems and the third costliest health condition in developed countries.
- It is the most common cause of adult disability in developed countries, requiring long term costly rehabilitation and is the principle cause of 1 out of every 16 deaths.
- For example, in Australia, a country with a population of less than 25 million, every 10 min someone has a stroke, and every 40 min, someone dies from one, with the total economic costs of stroke have been estimated to exceed $4 billion a year.
- The majority of strokes are ischemic in nature with only about 15% being due to haemorrhagic events.
- In ischemic stroke, a core area of tissue dies due to under-perfusion and an area of surrounding hypo-perfused tissue with patent collateral vessels remains salvageable. This hypo-perfused tissue has been referred to as the "penumbra" which if revascularised in a timely manner can be saved.
- In a typical acute ischemic stroke, the brain loses 1.9 million neurons, 14 billion synapses, and 7.5 miles of myelinated nerve fibres every minute.
- Therefore, urgent recanalisation of the occluded artery and restoration of blood flow is considered the most important therapeutic step to reperfuse threatened brain parenchyma before an irreversible infarction is established, to reduce morbidity and mortality.

H. Asadi, MD, PhD, FRANZCR, CCINR, EBIR
Interventional Neuroradiology Service, Austin Health, Melbourne, Victoria, Australia

School of Medicine, Faculty of Health, Deakin University, Victoria, Australia
e-mail: hamed.asadi@austin.org.au

H.K. Kok et al. (eds.), *Interventional Radiology for Medical Students*,
DOI 10.1007/978-3-319-53853-2_22

- Studies have estimated that there is a benefit of 1.8 days of added healthy life for each minute saved in terms of time to treatment, and a metanalysis has demonstrated that successful recanalisation increases the chance of a good functional outcome with an odds ratio of approximately 4.5, significantly reducing mortality at 3 months.

22.1.1 Treatment Options

22.1.1.1 Extra-Arterial Thrombolysis

- Almost 20 years ago, in 1996, intravenous tissue Plasminogen Activator (IV-tPA) was approved as the first thrombolysis medication and practically the only treatment option in ischemic strokes, when administered within 3 h from onset; Now, it is the standard first line treatment in those who are eligible (non-contrast CT brain excluding a haemorrhagic stroke).
- Provided no contraindications exist, it is administered at a dose of 0.9 mg/kg, with a maximum of 90 mg, with 10% of the medication given as a bolus and the remainder infused over 1 h.
- The safety and efficacy of IV-tPA within the first 3 h of the onset of symptoms was demonstrated in the NINDS (National Institute of Neurological Disorders and Stroke) study.
- However, the envelope of time limitation was stretched in subsequent research studies, like ECASS-3 (European Cooperative Acute Stroke Study 3), with the proposed guidelines changed accordingly to include those patients who presented within 4.5 h, and there is now an ever increasing number of trials looking into the safety and efficacy of IV-tPA beyond this time window.
- The success rate of IV-tPA in recanalisation is reduced in large vessel occlusion (thrombus in a major artery such as the internal carotid or middle cerebral arteries) and has never shown to be more than 50% and is more likely to be around 30%.
- This limited success in recanalisation, with critical time limitations, makes IV-tPA less than ideal in managing patients with large vessel occlusion.
- Overall, the success of intravenous thrombolysis depends on numerous factors including thrombus type, location and extent, collateral circulation, underlying comorbidities, patient's age, time to commencement of treatment and time to recanalisation; furthermore, studies have shown that large calibre proximal arteries are unlikely to be responsive to IV thrombolysis alone.
- Clinical trials have also shown that the likelihood of recanalisation negatively correlates with thrombus burden, with those having a clot size more than 8 mm in length having a significantly lower chance of achieving recanalisation by IV-tPA alone.
- The effectiveness of IV-tPA is also affected by the composition of the occlusive clot with emboli originated from large vessel atherosclerotic lesions (usually from the internal carotid artery) shown to be less responsive, compared with fibrin rich cardioembolic thombi.

- In addition, early reocclusion of arteries with large vessel occlusion has been shown to occur in up to 20% of cases, when recanalised initially by IV-tPA. Therefore, there have been major initiatives over the last several years to examine and develop new techniques to improve recanalisation rates and clinical outcome in patients with large vessel occlusion.
- These newly proposed therapeutic techniques not only consist of other extra-arterial methods of thrombolysis, but also a variety of endovascular techniques with the aim of improving revascularisation rates and improved clinical outcome.
- Endovascular techniques imply using a device which is inserted through the femoral artery in the groin to rapidly remove large vessel thrombus

22.1.1.2 Endovascular Treatment

- PROACT II (Prolyse in Acute Cerebral Thromboembolism) was the first study to examine the efficacy of intraarterial thrombolysis instead of intravenous thrombolysis, and since then intraarterial thrombolysis and mechanical thrombectomy has always had the appealing potential of rapid recanalisation and accelerated reperfusion with a potential for reduced haemorrhagic risk.
- The MERCI device was a corkscrew shape device with helical Nitinol loops, which was specifically designed for placement into the thrombus for enbloc removal. It was the first officially approved thrombectomy device with its safety and feasibility assessed in MERCI and Multi-MERCI trials.
- However, the idea of using stents in the treatment of acute ischemic stroke followed from the introduction of intracranial self-expanding stents for treatment of intracranial atherosclerotic stenosis.
- The initial attempts made in the treatment of acute ischemic stroke was by deployment of the stent across the thrombus at the occluded segment.
- One of the major conceivable complicating factors of this therapy was the need for concurrent antiplatelet-anticoagulation therapy and potential risk of haemorrhage.
- On the other hand, the introduction of detachable stents for stent assisted coiling of cerebral aneurysms, raised the possibility of using retrievable stents, which would retrieve clot in mechanical intracranial thrombectomy, with the further advantage of rapid recanalisation without the above-mentioned risks and complications of leaving a permanent stent in situ.
- The first two devices to be approved for this purpose were Solitaire-FR™ from Covidien® and Trevo™ from Stryker®, which were followed by similar products including Trevo-ProVUE™ (Stryker®), Revive™ (Johnson & Johnson®), EmboTrap™ (Neuravi®), Eric™ (Microvention®), Catch™ and Catch-Mini™ (Balt®).
- Contrary to suction thrombectomy or even stent insertion, these devices not only displace the thrombus to the periphery of the vessel and temporarily restore the flow, they also capture the thrombus by incorporating the clot through their interstices to make it possible to withdraw the trapped clot when the stent is removed.
- Following multiple initial futile attempts to prove the efficacy of mechanical thrombectomy, eventually in the second half of 2014 the Dutch MR-CLEAN

(Multicenter Randomized CLinical trial of Endovascular treatment for Acute ischemic stroke in the Netherlands) study demonstrated superiority in endovascular intervention, when the trial results were presented at the 9th World Stroke Congress.

- This was followed by release of the results of multiple other concurrent trials from around the world, including EXTEND-IA (Extending the Time for Thrombolysis in Emergency Neurological Deficits - Intra-Arterial) and ESCAPE (Endovascular treatment for Small Core And Proximal occlusion ischaemic stroke) which were very notably positive.
- Overall, these randomised control clinical trials were successful in demonstrating significant improvement in the outcome of patients with large vessel occlusion who received mechanical thrombectomy with decreased mortality when compared to the control groups who received IV thrombolysis.
- However, it is important to remember that even this endovascular treatment has a certain window of time and each one of the trials established a strict time window eligibility from the time of onset, with none of the patients enrolled undergoing endovascular mechanical thrombectomy more than 12 h from the time of onset of the stroke.

22.2 Procedure Indications

There is almost no consensus on indications for endovascular stroke intervention, and it is decided very much based on individual merits; however, the following are some of the important considerations:

- Severe stroke, with high stroke score. Depending on the centre, this is usually considered as NIHSS of more than 6. National Institute of Health Stroke Score (NIHSS) is a complicated, but validated and structured examination algorithm, commonly used to standardise assessment of the severity of stroke based on a scoring system (Table 22.1).
- Limited deficit but with significant impact on the victim, although NIHSS is low, e.g. aphasia in a young patient.
- Technical and expertise availability.
- Long segment proximal occlusion.
- Severe cervical arterial disease which needs concurrent treatment.
- Cervical arterial dissection which limits distal flow, requiring treatment.
- Unresponsiveness or contraindication to IV thrombolysis with tPA.
- Normal or near normal in usual daily activities, which can be assessed by ADL (Activities of Daily Living), but more commonly is measured by mRS (modified Rankin Score), and usually considered appropriate for intervention if mRS < 3 (Table 22.2).
- Posterior circulation stroke. Vertebrobasilar syndrome due to arterio-occlusive disease.

Table 22.1 Simplified and summarised version of NIHSS

Axis			Definition and scoring
Consciousness	1a. Level		0 = Alert; keenly responsive 1 = Not alert; but arousable by minor stimulation 2 = Not alert; requires repeated stimulation to attend 3 = Only reflexive/autonomic motor or unresponsive
	1b. Questions		0 = Answers both questions correctly 1 = Answers one question correctly 2 = Answers neither question correctly
	1c. Commands		0 = Performs both tasks correctly 1 = Performs one task correctly 2 = Performs neither task correctly
Eyes	2. Best gaze		0 = Normal 1 = Partial gaze palsy 2 = Forced deviation, or total gaze paresis not
	3. Visual		0 = No visual loss 1 = Partial hemianopia 2 = Complete hemianopia 3 = Bilateral hemianopia (including cortical)
Motor	4. Facial palsy:		0 = Normal symmetrical movements 1 = Minor paralysis 2 = Partial paralysis 3 = Complete paralysis
	5. Motor arm	5b. Right arm	0 = No drift 1 = Drift 2 = Some effort against gravity 3 = No effort against gravity 4 = No movement UN = Amputation or joint fusion
		5a. Left arm	
	6. Motor leg	6b. Right leg	0 = No drift 1 = Drift 2 = Some effort against gravity 3 = No effort against gravity 4 = No movement UN = Amputation or joint fusion
		6a. Left leg	
	7. Ataxia	Upper	0 = Absent 1 = Present in one limb 2 = Present in two limbs UN = Amputation or joint fusion
		Lower	
8. Sensory			0 = Normal; no sensory loss 1 = Mild-to-moderate sensory loss 2 = Severe to total sensory loss

(continued)

Table 22.1 (continued)

Axis		Definition and scoring
Speech	9. Best language	0 = No aphasia; normal 1 = Mild-to-moderate aphasia 2 = Severe aphasia 3 = Mute, global aphasia
	10. Dysarthria	0 = Normal 1 = Mild-to-moderate dysarthria 2 = Severe dysarthria UN = Intubated or other physical barrier
11. Extinction and inattention (neglect)		0 = No abnormality 1 = Sensory or personal inattention 2 = Profound hemi-inattention or extinction

Table 22.2 Simplified and summarised version of modified Rankin Scale (mRS) and Barthel index of Activities of Daily Living (ADL)

modified Rankin Scale	
mRS	Clinical status
0	No symptoms
1	No significant disability
2	Slight disability
3	Moderate disability, but able to walk
4	Moderately severe disability
5	Severe disability
6	Dead

Barthel index	
Axis	Condition
Incontinence	Faecal
	Urinary
Assistance needed with	Grooming
	Toilet use
	Feeding
	Transfers
	Walking
	Dressing
	Climbing stairs
	Bathing

22.3 Procedure Contraindications

It is always difficult not to treat a stroke victim, but the following should be considered as endovascular intervention may be fruitless and potentially harmful to the patient:

- Lack of expertise or unavailability of the required technology.
- Large established infarction at the time of presentation, based on CT/MR perfusion or diffusion studies. The exact volume differs depending on the institutional experience, but generally greater than 70–100 ml of infarction core.
- Large infarction core based on the noncontrast CT brain.
- Proven absence of significant amount of salvageable tissue. This depends on the availability of advanced penumbral imaging (using special CT or MR techniques) and local expertise.
- Very late presentation (usually more than 6–8 h post onset), or a wakeup-stroke (someone who was likely asleep when stroke happened).
- However, patients who present late, but do not have a large infarction core, may still benefit from intervention. This depends on the individual institutional policy.
- Advanced comorbidities with poor prognosis, or advanced disability, with low ADL and usually mRS > 3.
- Presence of intracranial hemorrhage.
- Inability to gain arterial access, due to vascular occlusion or tortuosity.
- Mild stroke with low NIH stroke score (NIHSS).
- Small distal vascular occlusion, as current evidence is limited to the large proximal arterial thromboembolic disease.

22.4 Patient Preparation

- In patients with large vessel occlusion as determined by CT, IV-tPA should not be delayed, and if indicated should be given immediately after a haemorrhagic stroke has been ruled out.
- If large vessel occlusion is seen a CT angiogram from aortic arch to the vertex of the skull is performed.
- Penumbral imaging (to estimate the size of the penumbra in patients with large vessel occlusion) and assessement of collateral pathways is performed depending on institutional availability.
- Immediate transfer to the angiographic suite, if no contraindications.
- Controlling the blood pressure above a certain level. The exact level depends on the institutional experience and the patient history of systemic hypertension, but generally a systolic blood pressure below 140 mmHg is likely detrimental.
- Preference is for intervention to be performed with the paient awake to avoid potential delay as well as any hypotension developing during induction of anesthesia. However, if the patient is very uncooperative, liaison with anesthesiology is needed.
- Conscious sedation if absolutely required.

- Prioritizing the activities in the angiography suite to avoid any delay, e.g. transportation, preparing the access site, or collecting required equipment.
- Blood tests, or correction of patient's coagulative status is generally not recommended, as can it delay revascularisation.

22.5 Complications

Overall, mechanical thrombectomy in a subspecialised center carries less than 12% risk, and although symptomatic intercranial haemorrhage is likely the most common complication post thrombectomy, seen in approximately 5% of the cases; it is unlikely to be solely related to the procedure itself and is most likely contributed to by naturally caused haemorrhagic transformation within the established infarction core.

- Intracranial arterial rupture.
- Clot fragmentation and distal arterial embolisation ('trashing').
- Failure to recanalise or partial revascularisation.
- Brain artery complications: dissection or severe vasospasm.
- Groin complications: dissection, occlusion, haemorrhage, and pseudoaneurysm.
- If cervical carotid recanalisation/stenting is also required: dissection, occlusion, stent failure or complications secondary to anticoagulation and antiplatelet.
- Death.

22.6 Case Study

22.6.1 Presentation

- Fifty-four-year-old female patient.
- She presented with stroke to a tertiary hospital at 3:30 pm.
- She had a collapse at home at around 1:30 pm, with persistent right facial droop, slurring of speech and right arm weakness at the time of presentation.
- The stroke score was estimated at 18 based on NIHSS at the time of presentation.
- In the history, patient was diagnosed with atrial fibrillation and was on warfarin until 10 days earlier when it was stopped prior to an elective mastectomy for breast cancer.
- Otherwise there was no significant clinical history with patient fully active and still working as a secretary (mRS of 0).

22.6.2 Imaging Investigation

- Initial CT brain demonstrated a long segment hyperdense thrombus in the MCA (middle cerebral artery) with moderate size established infarction, involving the left frontal and temporal lobes, as well as the insular ribbon.

- On the CT angiogram, the left ICA (internal carotid artery) was not opacified beyond its middle third, with an occluded intracranial ICA.
- MCA was occluded with multiphase CTA demonstrating good collateral perfusion to the affected territories.

22.6.3 Management and Procedure

- Because the mastectomy surgery was performed only 3 days earlier, after quick consultation with the surgeon, the decision was made not to administer thrombolysis with IV-tPA and after discussion with the interventional neuroradiologist, the patient was transferred to a comprehensive stroke center for endovascular thrombectomy.
- After arrival to the angiographic suite, a right CFA 8Fr uphill access was established followed by a left carotid angiogram. The ICA opacified to its supra-ophthalmic portion, with a stagnant column of contrast, indicating a further distal occlusion (Fig. 22.1).
- An 8Fr guidecatheter was placed within the distal cervical ICA, followed by insertion of an intermediate catheter into the petrosal ICA.
- A small microcatheter with a microwire were advanced through the occluded MCA and placed into the inferior MCA division, with the position confirmed using small amounts of contrast material.

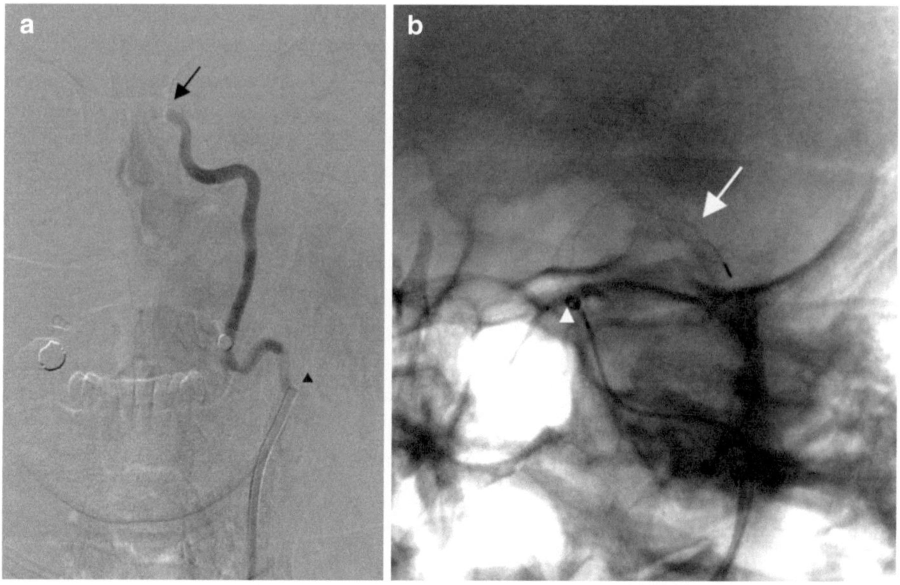

Fig. 22.1 (**a**) Left ICA frontal angiograms with the tip of the guidecatheter (*Arrow head*) at the carotid bulb, demonstrating no luminal opacification beyond the supra-ophthalmic segment (*Arrow*). (**b**) An intermediate catheter was placed into the petrosal ICA, then an inner microcatheter/microwire (*Arrowhead*) was advanced through the occluded MCA and a stentretriever was placed across the occluded segment of the artery (*Arrow*)

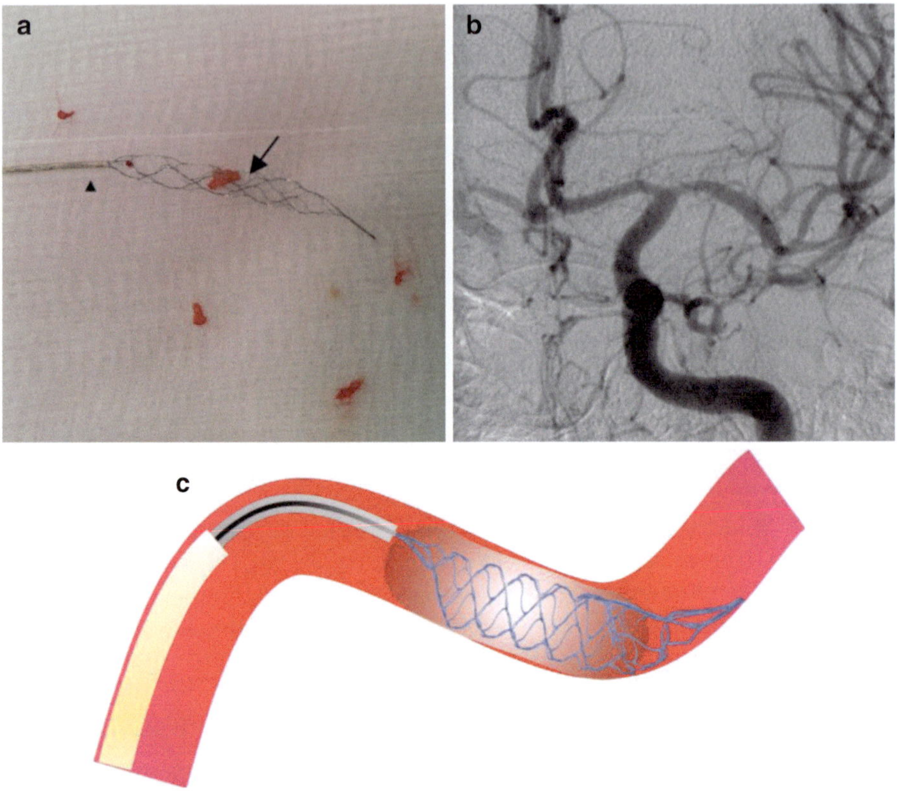

Fig. 22.2 (**a**) Stentretriever (*Arrow*) and microcatheter (*Arrow head*) were withdrawn together with small thromboembolic fragments extracted. (**b**) Complete MCA recanalisation with normal opacification of the distal branches. (**c**) Schematic diagram demonstrating positioning of the guidecatheter (*Yellow*), microcatheter (*Grey*) and stentretriever (*Blue* with *Black* Pusher) relative to the thrombus (*Brown*) within the Artery (*Red*)

- Subsequently a stentretriever was advanced through the microcatheter with its distal portion and the leading tip parked beyond the thrombus (Fig. 22.2).
- The stent not only pushes the thrombus against the wall of the artery, but also thrombus passes through the relatively large interstices of the stent, and is trapped inside.
- After a 3–5 min delay, the stent-retriever and microcatheter were withdrawn while vigorous suction was applied through the guidecatheter.
- Moderate amounts of thromboemboli were extracted with complete recanalisation of the MCA and its inferior division.
- Stentretriever was then placed within the superior division, and further thromboembolic fragments were extracted.
- Complete recanalisation of the MCA and its divisions demonstrated on the final runs at 5:30 pm, approximately 4 h post stroke onset (Fig. 22.2).

22.6.4 Outcome

- Patient was transferred back to the referring hospital with significant clinical improvement within the course of the next 24 h with a final stroke score of 5, improved from 18.

22.7 Post-procedure Care and Review

- Post-operatively patients are usually transferred to a high dependency or neuro-intensive unit depending on their clinical status for close monitoring of clinical status and vital parameters, e.g. BP.
- If the procedure is performed under general anesthesia, they will be transferred to a dedicated recovery area.
- All immediate post-procedure patients require regular monitoring of the arterial puncture site and limb vascular assessment.
- Regular neurological assessment, as per institutional protocol.
- Patients with acute ischemic stroke usually remain as inpatient for at least 2–3 days depending on their recovery, followed by rehabilitations if needed. Those who need further investigations for the cause of stroke will stay longer.
- There is no universal consensus regarding post-procedure followup, but a repeat CT in 24 h is recommended to assess for the size of established infarction, and to exclude potential haemorrhagic transformation prior to commencement of anti-coagulation or antiplatelet medication if indicated.

22.8 Case Discussion

- Acute ischemic stroke (AIS) is a serious medical condition, with a high morbidity and mortality, as well as large social and economic impact.
- The clinical severity of a victim of acute ischemic stroke is usually measured based on a complex clinical scoring system introduced by the National Institutes of Health in the USA (NIHSS) (Table 22.1).
- The patient's abilities in terms of day to day activities is estimated using a scoring system developed by Glascow University and subsequently modified by the researchers at the University of Edinburgh, mRS (modified Rankin Score) (Table 22.2)
- The aim in treating acute ischemic stroke is to recanalise the occluded artery, revascularise the affected territory and ultimately reperfuse salvageable tissue before the infarction core progresses further.
- Revascularisation can be achieved by using intravenous thrombolytic agents; however, they have limited success in patienst with large vessel thrombus/occlusion and combined endovascular treatment with thrombolysis, if possible, has been shown to be superior in these patients with large vessel occlusion.

- Stentretrievers have revolutionised endovascular recanalisation with more than an 85% success rate; however, not all thromboemboli are extractable and sometimes other techniques, including suction thrombectomy may be required.

Key Points

- Acute stroke is a relatively common clinical condition, requiring emergency treatment, with potential for significant morbidity and mortality.
- The most common type of stroke is ischemic in nature (more than 85%), compared with haemorrhagic stroke (approximately 15%).
- Urgent revascularisation of the occluded artery is the primary goal in management of acute ischemic stroke.
- Intravenous thrombolysis with tPA has been the standard treatment for those presented with AIS for the last two decades, and is still of great therapeutic value.
- However, some patients have contraindications for IV thrombolysis, and in addition, it has been shown to be ineffective in treating major arterial occlusions with large clot burden.
- Following the recent randomised controlled trials, endovascular thrombectomy is becoming the standard treatment in managing AIS with large arterial occlusion.
- Overall, no matter what technique is adopted in treating ischemic stroke victims, the ultimate goal is to reperfuse the threatened salvageable brain parenchyma as soon as possible to minimise the size of final infarction core and hence its clinical consequences.

Suggested Reading

1. Albers GW, Amarenco P, Easton JD, Sacco RL, Teal P. Antithrombotic and thrombolytic therapy for ischemic stroke: the Seventh ACCP Conference on Antithrombotic and Thrombolytic Therapy. Chest. 2004;126(3 Suppl):483S–512S. Epub 2004/09/24.
2. Asadi H, Dowling R, Yan B, Wong S, Mitchell P. Advances in endovascular treatment of acute ischemic stroke. Intern Med J. 2014;45(8):798–805.
3. Asadi H, Yan B, Dowling R, Wong S, Mitchell P. Advances in medical revascularisation treatments in acute ischemic stroke. Thrombosis. 2014;2014:714218.
4. Barreto AD, Alexandrov AV. Adjunctive and alternative approaches to current reperfusion therapy. Stroke. 2012;43(2):591–8. Epub 2012/01/10.
5. Blackham KA, Meyers PM, Abruzzo TA, Albuquerque FC, Fiorella D, Fraser J, et al. Endovascular therapy of acute ischemic stroke: report of the standards of practice Committee of the Society of NeuroInterventional surgery. J Neurointerv Surg. 2012;4(2):87–93. Epub 2012/01/27.
6. Choi K-E, Hall CL, Sun J-M, Wei L, Mohamad O, Dix TA, et al. A novel stroke therapy of pharmacologically induced hypothermia after focal cerebral ischemia in mice. FASEB J. 2012;26(7):2799–810.

7. del Zoppo GJ, Poeck K, Pessin MS, Wolpert SM, Furlan AJ, Ferbert A, et al. Recombinant tissue plasminogen activator in acute thrombotic and embolic stroke. Ann Neurol. 1992;32(1):78–86. Epub 1992/07/01.
8. Del Zoppo GJ, Saver JL, Jauch EC, Adams HP Jr. Expansion of the time window for treatment of acute ischemic stroke with intravenous tissue plasminogen activator: a science advisory from the American Heart Association/American Stroke Association. Stroke. 2009;40(8):2945–8. Epub 2009/05/30.
9. Eissa A, Krass I, Levi C, Sturm J, Ibrahim R, Bajorek B. Understanding the reasons behind the low utilisation of thrombolysis in stroke. Australas Med J. 2013;6(3):152.
10. Ferrell AS, Britz GW. Developments on the horizon in the treatment of neurovascular problems. Surg Neurol Int. 2013;4(Suppl 1):S31–7. Epub 2013/05/09.
11. Fiorella DJ, Levy EI, Turk AS, Albuquerque FC, Pride GL Jr, Woo HH, et al. Target lesion revascularization after wingspan: assessment of safety and durability. Stroke. 2009;40(1):106–10. Epub 2008/10/18.
12. Fitzsimmons B-F, Becske T, Nelson P. Rapid stent-supported revascularization in acute ischemic stroke. Am J Neuroradiol. 2006;27(5):1132–4.
13. Fulkerson J, Ferrera DA, Cragg A. Acute stroke revascularization/recanalization systems processes and products thereby. Google Patents; 2009.
14. Gonzalez RG, Copen WA, Schaefer PW, Lev MH, Pomerantz SR, Rapalino O, et al. The Massachusetts General Hospital acute stroke imaging algorithm: an experience and evidence based approach. J Neurointerv Surg. 2013;5(Suppl 1):i7–12. Epub 2013/03/16.
15. Hacke W, Kaste M, Bluhmki E, Brozman M, Davalos A, Guidetti D, et al. Thrombolysis with alteplase 3 to 4.5 hours after acute ischemic stroke. N Engl J Med. 2008;359(13):1317–29. Epub 2008/09/26.
16. Levy EI, Mehta R, Gupta R, Hanel RA, Chamczuk AJ, Fiorella D, et al. Self-expanding stents for recanalization of acute cerebrovascular occlusions. AJNR Am J Neuroradiol. 2007;28(5):816–22. Epub 2007/05/15.
17. Majid A. Neuroprotection in stroke: past, present, and future. ISRN Neurol. 2014;2014:515716.
18. Meretoja A, Keshtkaran M, Saver JL, Tatlisumak T, Parsons MW, Kaste M, et al. Stroke thrombolysis save a minute, save a day. Stroke. 2014;45(4):1053–8.
19. Molina CA, Montaner J, Arenillas JF, Ribo M, Rubiera M, Alvarez-Sabín J. Differential pattern of tissue plasminogen activator-induced proximal middle cerebral artery recanalization among stroke subtypes. Stroke (A Journal of Cerebral Circulation). 2004;35(2):486–90.
20. National Institute of Neurological Disorders and Stroke rt-PA Stroke Study Group. Tissue plasminogen activator for acute ischemic stroke. N Engl J Med. 1995;333(24):1581–7.
21. Nogueira RG, Schwamm LH, Buonanno FS, Koroshetz WJ, Yoo AJ, Rabinov JD, et al. Low-pressure balloon angioplasty with adjuvant pharmacological therapy in patients with acute ischemic stroke caused by intracranial arterial occlusions. Neuroradiology. 2008;50(4):331–40. Epub 2008/01/04.
22. Penumbra Pivotal Stroke Trial Investigators. The penumbra pivotal stroke trial: safety and effectiveness of a new generation of mechanical devices for clot removal in intracranial large vessel occlusive disease. Stroke. 2009;40(8):2761–8. Epub 2009/07/11.
23. Rha JH, Saver JL. The impact of recanalization on ischemic stroke outcome: a meta-analysis. Stroke. 2007;38(3):967–73.
24. Riedel CH, Zimmermann P, Jensen-Kondering U, Stingele R, Deuschl G, Jansen O. The importance of size: successful recanalization by intravenous thrombolysis in acute anterior stroke depends on thrombus length. Stroke. 2011;42(6):1775–7. Epub 2011/04/09.
25. Rubiera M, Alvarez-Sabín J, Ribo M, Montaner J, Santamarina E, Arenillas JF, et al. Predictors of early arterial reocclusion after tissue plasminogen activator-induced recanalization in acute ischemic stroke. Stroke. 2005;36(7):1452–6.

26. Saqqur M, Uchino K, Demchuk AM, Molina CA, Garami Z, Calleja S, et al. Site of arterial occlusion identified by transcranial Doppler predicts the response to intravenous thrombolysis for stroke. Stroke. 2007;38(3):948–54. Epub 2007/02/10.
27. Saver JL, Jahan R, Levy EI, Jovin TG, Baxter B, Nogueira RG, et al. Solitaire flow restoration device versus the Merci Retriever in patients with acute ischaemic stroke (SWIFT): a randomised, parallel-group, non-inferiority trial. Lancet. 2012;380(9849):1241–9. Epub 2012/08/31.
28. Smith WS, Sung G, Saver J, Budzik R, Duckwiler G, Liebeskind DS, et al. Mechanical thrombectomy for acute ischemic stroke: final results of the Multi MERCI trial. Stroke. 2008;39(4):1205–12. Epub 2008/03/01.
29. Smith WS, Sung G, Starkman S, Saver JL, Kidwell CS, Gobin YP, et al. Safety and efficacy of mechanical embolectomy in acute ischemic stroke: results of the MERCI trial. Stroke. 2005;36(7):1432–8. Epub 2005/06/18.

Aneurysmal Subarachnoid Hemorrhage (aSAH)

23

Hamed Asadi

23.1 Introduction

- The overall prevalence of cerebral aneurysms has been reported variably from 3.6% to 6% of the worldwide population, translating to approximately 1 in 50 people having an unruptured aneurysm in the United States.
- They are most prevalent at 35–60 years of age with newly diagnosed aneurysms mostly developing in patient's older than 40.
- Paediatric cases are also diagnosed, mainly in the context of underlying syndromic conditions.
- There is a slight female predilection for aneurysms with a female to male ratio of approximately 3–2.
- The majority of the aneurysms measure between 3 and 2.5 cm in diameter (65–85%) and carry a low-rupture risk (less than or equal to 1% per year).
- Aneurysms larger than 2.5 cm are referred to as "Giant". Ten to 15% of patients diagnosed with a cerebral aneurysm have another aneurysm.

23.1.1 Aneurysm Rupture

- Rupture of cerebral aneurysms, also known as aneurysmal subarachnoid haemorrhage (aSAH), is a significant cause of death and disability worldwide, estimated at half a million deaths every year, with approximately 40% overall mortality; however, an estimated 50 to 80 percent of all aneurysms never rupture or cause any symptoms during a person's lifetime.

H. Asadi, MD, PhD, FRANZCR, CCINR, EBIR
Interventional Neuroradiology Service, Austin Health, Melbourne, Victoria, Australia

School of Medicine, Faculty of Health, Deakin University, Victoria, Australia
e-mail: hamed.asadi@austin.org.au

H.K. Kok et al. (eds.), *Interventional Radiology for Medical Students*,
DOI 10.1007/978-3-319-53853-2_23

- On the contrary, large and in particular, giant aneurysms can pose a significant risk of complications, with the annual rate of rupture estimated to be 6–12 or more precisely 8–10 per 100,000 people, equating to 30,000 patients in the United States per year, or approximately one aneurysm rupture every 18 min. Overall, giant aneurysms have more than 40% risk of rupture over 5 years.
- The median age of aneurysmal rupture is 50 years of age, with typically no warning signs, and it accounts for approximately 3–5% of all new strokes within the whole population.

23.1.2 Outcome of Subarachnoid Haemorrhage (SAH)

- About 10–15% of patients with aneurysmal haemorrhage will die before reaching hospital with a subsequent 25% mortality within the first 24 h of the hemorrhage.
- The overall survival rate is estimated at less than 50%.
- Amongst survivors, approximately 66% suffer a permanent neurological deficit, while approximately 4 out of 7 people who recover from a ruptured brain aneurysm will have long-term disabilities.
- A study in 2004 estimated the combined financial impact of these survivors and their carers, as up to $138,000,000 annually in the United States alone.
- Not only is there a high morbidity and mortality associated with aneurysm rupture, but also aneurysm treatment costs significantly increase after a rupture.

23.1.3 Treatment

- The ultimate goal in treating an unruptured intracranial aneurysm is to exclude it from the circulation to prevent rupture.
- However, if an aneurysm has already bled, it still needs to be secured to prevent rebleeding.
- Prior to the introduction of the Guglielmi detachable coils (GDC) in 1990, making endovascular coiling of the aneurysms possible, the only treatment option available was open surgical clipping.
- Advances in equipment and techniques, including invention of three dimensional coils, micro-stents and balloons as well as flow divertor stents, parallel to the introduction of balloon and stent assisted coiling, have made endovascular treatment of wide neck or dissecting aneurysms possible.
- Endovascular intervention is now considered the first line treatment for intracranial aneurysms, after results from the International Subarachnoid Aneurysmal Trial (ISAT) showed that endovascular coiling was associated with lower morbidity and mortality rates compared with neurosurgical clipping.
- The optimal timing of definitive management for acutely ruptured intracranial aneurysms has been the subject of considerable debate over the last few decades.
- Although it was always believed that early treatment decreases the risk of rebleeding, is was historically regarded as a higher risk than a delayed procedure.

- However, over time there has been a move from the advocacy of "late intervention", defined as more than 10 days post aneurysmal rupture, towards "early" surgery, defined as one to 3 days post SAH; and even recently a few studies have proposed "ultra-early" intervention, defined as within 24 h post SAH with improved clinical outcome.

23.1.4 Long-Term Prognosis

- Overall trends show that survival rates are increasing, despite the fact that the incidence of aSAH appears to be largely unchanged.
- However, because of all the advances in the management of aneurysms and post procedural care, there is an ever increasing number of people surviving who are potentially left with serious physical and cognitive deficits associated with significant financial burden and reduced quality of life.
- Additionally, there are increasing numbers of patients with coiled aneurysms; requiring clinical and imaging follow up for early detection of aneurysm recurrence or recanalisation.

23.2 Procedure Indications

- Aneurysmal subarachnoid hemorrhage (Aneurysm Rupture).
- Unruptured aneurysm with estimated high risk for future rupture.
- Previously treated aneurysms (ruptured or unruptured) with significant recanalisation.
- Previously treated aneurysms (ruptured or unruptured) with significant recurrence.
- Aneurysms associated with other intracranial vascular anomalies (e.g. AVMs) with high risk of haemorrhage.
- Extradural Aneurysms (no risk for SAH) which are complicated (e.g. cranial neuropathy due to mass effect).

23.3 Procedure Contraindications

There is almost no absolute contraindication in treating a ruptured cerebral aneurysm endovascularly; however, some relative contraindications are usually considered:

- Lack of expertise or unavailability of the required technology.
- Extremely poor prognosis, in particular clinical or imaging evidence for extensive irreversible brain injuries.
- Severe comorbidities with very poor overall outcome.
- Extensive intraparenchymal haemorrhage with mass effect, requiring emergency urgent craniotomy and evacuation, in particular if the aneurysm is in the vicinity of the surgical field and amenable to clipping at the time of surgery.

- Technical difficulty, either due to aneurysm morphology or vascular access.
- If endovascular treatment is only possible by insertion of scaffolding devices (e.g. stents), and anticoagulation or antiplatelet therapy is contraindicated.

23.4 Patient Preparation

For patients with ruptured aneurysm and subarachnoid haemorrhage:

- Thorough neurological assessment.
- Start fasting with anaesthetics review.
- Routine blood investigations.
- Optimisation of the coagulation profile if technically possible (preferably INR < 1.5 and PLTs >50,000).
- Reversal of potential anticoagulation or antiplatelets, if clinically possible.
- Insertion of ventricular drains if urgently necessary for hydrocephalus.
- Medical management of increased intracranial pressure if necessary.
- Vasospasm prophylaxis treatment as per institutional protocol (e.g. Nimodipine infusion-dihydropyridine calcium channel blocker).
- Blood pressure control based as per institutional protocols (e.g. mean arterial pressure < 130 mmHg), preferably with agents which have no detrimental effects on the intracranial pressure.
- Premedication, based on individual institutional protocols, if there is any history of significant contrast medium reactions.

23.5 Complications

Overall, complications are more likely in the case of a ruptured aneurysm compared with elective procedures:

- On table aneurysm rupture.
- On table parent artery rupture.
- Infarction due to: thromboembolism, coil protrusion or arterial sacrifice.
- Stent complications: occlusion, thromboembolism, and stenosis.
- Access complications: dissection or severe vasospasm.
- Balloon complications: dissection, rupture and thrombosis.
- Groin complications: dissection, occlusion, haemorrhage, and pseudoaneurysm.
- Death.

23.6 Case Study

- Fifty-five-year-old female patient.
- Presented with severe headache and progressive confusion.

- This was diagnosed as subarachnoid haemorrhage on a noncontract CT brain.
- After informed consent from the next of kin, with aseptic technique while under general anaesthesia, via a right CFA uphill 8 French access, bilateral ICA and vertebral DSA (Digital Subtraction Angiography) was performed.
- DSA demonstrated a right MCA bifurcation saccular aneurysm measuring approximately 3 mm × 3 mm in perpendicular dimensions, with the neck estimated to be 3 mm wide (Fig. 23.1).
- After the configuration of the aneurysm was further assessed using a 3D reconstructed image (Fig. 23.2) and deemed to be amenable for endovascular

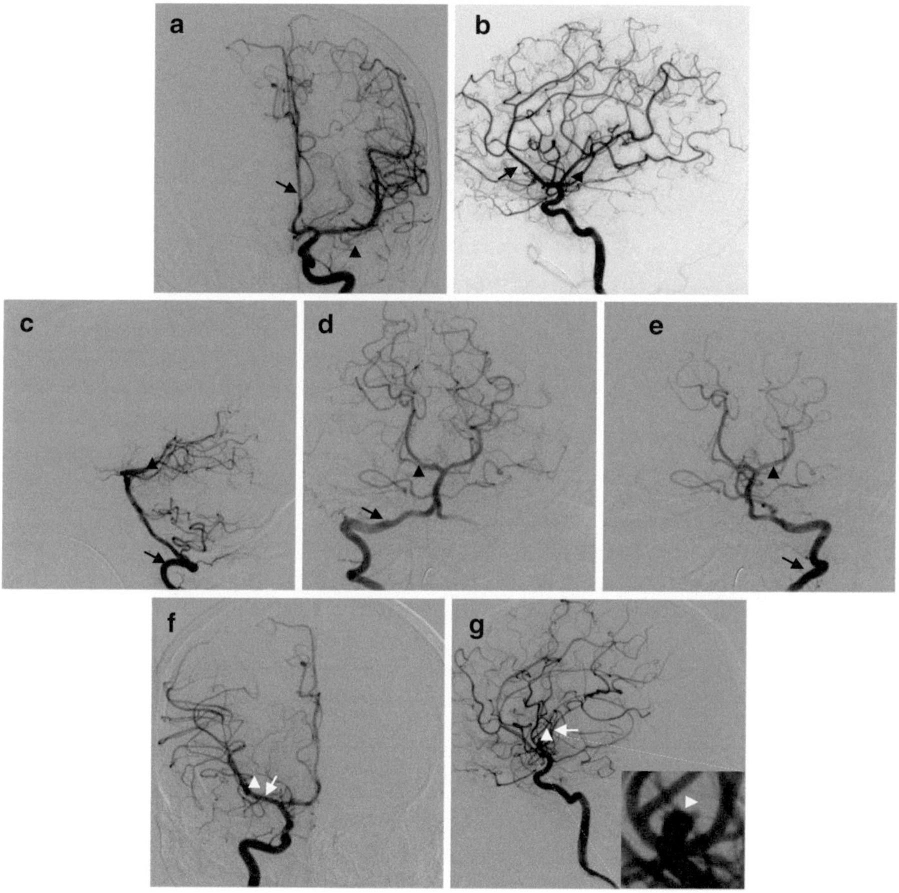

Fig. 23.1 Left ICA frontal (**a**) and lateral (**b**) angiograms (*Arrow*: ACA, *Arrowhead*: MCA & its branches), as well as lateral (**c**) and frontal (**d**) right and frontal (**e**) left vertebrobasilar injections (*Arrow*: right and left vertebral, *Arrowhead*: right and left PCAs), demonstrating normal anatomy with no aneurysms or significant vasospasm. Right ICA injection confirmed presence of a relatively small MCA bifurcation aneurysm (*Arrow*: right MCA & its branches, Arrowhead: bifurcation aneurysm), on both frontal (**f**) and lateral (**g**) projections (with magnified view of the aneurysm)

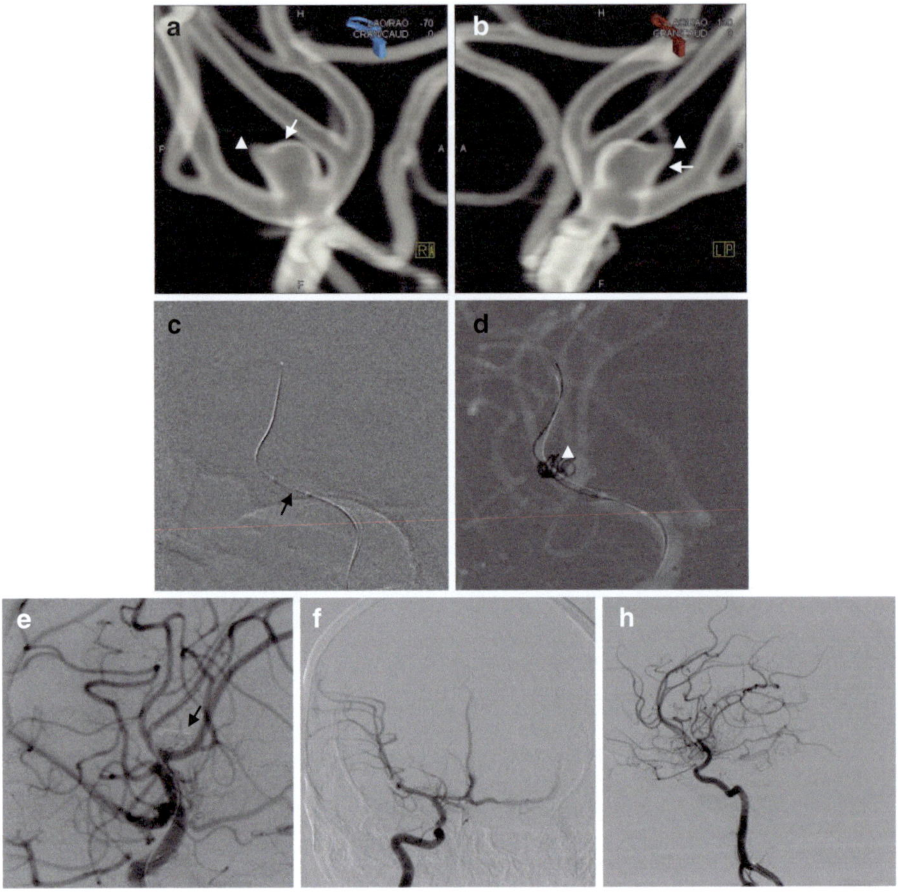

Fig. 23.2 External (**a**) and internal (**b**) rotational projections of the 3D surface rendered right MCA bifurcation aneurysm (*Arrow*) for operational planning, demonstrating its saccular configuration and position of the neck, as well as likely point of rupture (*Arrow head*) Then a balloon (Hyperform) was positioned across the aneurysm neck (*Arrow*) and the aneurysm was coil embolised (*Arrow head*) through a microcatheter (Courier) (**c** and **d**). Good packing of the aneurysm (*Arrow*) with no complications (**e**, **f** and **g**)

treatment, the aneurysm was treated by balloon-assisted coiling (Fig. 23.2) with good exclusion of the aneurysm from the circulation.

- During the operation, 7000 international units of heparin was administered to prevent potential thromboembolic events.

23.7 Post-procedure Care and Review

- Post-operatively patients are usually transferred to a recovery bay following general anaesthesia.
- Decision regarding extubation depends on the patients' clinical status.

- Patients with a low GCS usually remain intubated and are reassessed for extubation depending on clinical progress.
- Patients with aSAH are transferred to ICU or HDU depending on their clinical status for close monitoring of clinical status and vital parameters, e.g. BP.
- Patients with aSAH remain on vasospasm-protective treatment, depending on institutional protocols, e.g. nimodipine for 10 days.
- All immediate post operative patients require regular monitoring of the arterial puncture site and limb vascular assessment, as per local protocol.
- All post operative patients require regular neurological assessment.
- aSAH patients should be rigorously monitored for development of vasospasm and if clinically suspicious may require further vascular imaging.
- Depending on the results of vasospasm investigation, further medical or endovascular interventions may be required.
- In cases requiring stent insertion, the patient may need loading or ongoing doses of antiplatelets or anticoagulation.
- Patients with aSAH usually remain as inpatients for at least 10 days to 2 weeks depending on their recovery followed by rehabilitations if needed.
- Uncomplicated elective cases are normally discharged in 24–48 h.
- There is no universal consensus regarding post-procedure followup, but as a rule of thumb, an endovascularly treated aneurysm should be revaluated in 3–6 months followed by annual imaging for 5 years to assess for recanalisation, recurrence or de novo new aneurysms. After 5 years, the interval is commonly changed to biannual follow-up.

23.8 Case Discussion

- Aneurysm rupture and subarachnoid hemorrhage is a serious medical condition, with high morbidity and mortality.
- The clinical severity of a victim of subarachnoid hemorrhage is usually graded based on the system introduced by World Federation of Neurological Societies (WFNS):

Grade	Clinical presentation
I	GCS 15
II	GCS 13–14 without deficit
III	GCS 13–14 with focal neurological deficit
IV	GCS 7–12
V	GCS < 7

- The size and extent of SAH is graded on noncontrast CT brain imaging.
- The aim in treating an aneurysm whether ruptured or unruptured is to exclude it from the circulation either externally, i.e. surgical clipping, or endovascularly.
- Endovascular treatment is achieved either by filling the aneurysm cavity or by covering its neck, to prevent entrance of blood into the aneurysmal sac.

- Endovascular treatment of aneurysms is performed under general anesthesia, mainly to avoid any potential movement of the head rather than due to the potential procedural discomfort.
- Coils are of different size, shapes and length and those used for cerebral embolisation are almost exclusively detachable.
- Overall, patients who undergo coil embolisation have a higher risk for recanalisation and must be followed with imaging.

Key Points

- Cerebral aneurysms are relatively common but rupture is comparatively rare.
- Cerebral aneurysm rupture usually leads to subarachnoid hemorrhage which is a very serious medical condition with high morbidity and mortality.
- Emergency specialised care is needed for those with SAH, and they should be managed by a multidisciplinary team.
- Treatment of the cerebral aneurysms can be performed by open surgical clipping, or by endovascular methods.
- Overall, endovascular treatment of aneurysms is the preferred technique with less morbidity and better outcome, however it depends on the technical suitability and availability of the technology and expertise.

Suggested Reading

1. Bowles E. Cerebral aneurysm and aneurysmal subarachnoid haemorrhage. Nurs Stand. 2014;28(34):52–9.
2. Cha KC, Kim JH, Kang HI, Moon BG, Lee SJ, Kim JS. Aneurysmal rebleeding: factors associated with clinical outcome in the rebleeding patients. J Korean Neurosurg Soc. 2010;47(2):119–23.
3. Chyatte D, Fode NC, Sundt TM Jr. Early versus late intracranial aneurysm surgery in subarachnoid hemorrhage. J Neurosurg. 1988;69(3):326–31.
4. Connolly PJ, Biller J, Pritz MB. Aneurysm observation versus intervention: a literature review. Neurol Res. 2002;24(Suppl 1):S84–95.
5. Foundation BA. Understanding: brain aneurysm statistics and facts. [cited; Available from: http://www.bafound.org/Statistics_and_Facts.
6. Guglielmi G, Viñuela F, Dion J, Duckwiler G. Electrothrombosis of saccular aneurysms via endovascular approach: Part 2: preliminary clinical experience. J Neurosurg. 1991;75(1):8–14.
7. Higashida RT, Smith W, Gress D, Urwin R, Dowd CF, Balousek PA, et al. Intravascular stent and endovascular coil placement for a ruptured fusiform aneurysm of the basilar artery: case report and review of the literature. J Neurosurg. 1997;87(6):944–9.
8. Ishibashi T, Murayama Y, Urashima M, Saguchi T, Ebara M, Arakawa H, et al. Unruptured intracranial aneurysms incidence of rupture and risk factors. Stroke (A Journal of Cerebral Circulation). 2009;40(1):313–6.
9. Juszkat R, Nowak S, Smol S, Kociemba W, Blok T, Zarzecka A. Leo Stent for endovascular treatment of broad-necked and fusiform intracranial aneurysms. Interv Neuroradiol

(Journal of Peritherapeutic Neuroradiology, Surgical Procedures and Related Neurosciences). 2007;13(3):255–69.
10. Juvela S, Porras M, Heiskanen O. Natural history of unruptured intracranial aneurysms: a long-term follow-up study. J Neurosurg. 1993;79(2):174–82.
11. Juvela S, Poussa K, Porras M. Factors affecting formation and growth of intracranial aneurysms a long-term follow-up study. Stroke (A Journal of Cerebral Circulation). 2001;32(2):485–91.
12. Laidlaw JD, Siu KH. Poor-grade aneurysmal subarachnoid hemorrhage: outcome after treatment with urgent surgery. Neurosurgery. 2003;53(6):1275–82.
13. Laidlaw JD, Siu KH. Ultra-early surgery for aneurysmal subarachnoid hemorrhage: outcomes for a consecutive series of 391 patients not selected by grade or age. J Neurosurg. 2002;97(2):250–8.
14. Ljunggren B, Säveland H, Brandt L. Causes of unfavorable outcome after early aneurysm operation. Neurosurgery. 1983;13(6):629–33.
15. Molyneux A. International subarachnoid aneurysm Trial (ISAT) collaborative group: international subarachnoid aneurysm Trial (ISAT) of neurosurgical clipping versus endovascular coiling in 2143 patients with ruptured intracranial aneurysms: a randomised comparison of effects on survival, dependency, seizures, rebleeding, subgroups, and aneurysm occlusion. Lancet. 2005;366(9488):809–17.
16. Nieuwkamp DJ, Setz LE, Algra A, Linn FH, de Rooij NK, Rinkel GJ. Changes in case fatality of aneurysmal subarachnoid haemorrhage over time, according to age, sex, and region: a meta-analysis. Lancet Neurol. 2009;8(7):635–42.
17. Pan J-W, Zhan R-Y, Wen L, Tong Y, Wan S, Zhou Y-Y. Ultra-early surgery for poor-grade intracranial aneurysmal subarachnoid hemorrhage: a preliminary study. Yonsei Med J. 2009;50(4):521–4.
18. Phatouros CC, Sasaki TY, Higashida RT, Malek AM, Meyers PM, Dowd CF, et al. Stent-supported coil embolization: the treatment of fusiform and wide-neck aneurysms and pseudoaneurysms. Neurosurgery. 2000;47(1):107–15.
19. Phillips TJ, Dowling RJ, Yan B, Laidlaw JD, Mitchell PJ. Does treatment of ruptured intracranial aneurysms within 24 hours improve clinical outcome? Stroke (A Journal of Cerebral Circulation). 2011;42(7):1936–45.
20. Roos Y, Beenen L, Groen R, Albrecht K, Vermeulen M. Timing of surgery in patients with aneurysmal subarachnoid haemorrhage: rebleeding is still the major cause of poor outcome in neurosurgical units that aim at early surgery. J Neurol Neurosurg Psychiatry. 1997;63(4):490–3.
21. Steiner T, Juvela S, Unterberg A, Jung C, Forsting M, Rinkel G. European stroke organization guidelines for the management of intracranial aneurysms and subarachnoid haemorrhage. Cerebrovasc Dis. 2013;35(2):93–112.
22. Wardlaw J, White P. The detection and management of unruptured intracranial aneurysms. Brain. 2000;123(2):205–21.
23. Wiebers D, Whisnant J, Huston J 3rd, Meissner I, Brown RD Jr, Piepgras DG, International Study of Unruptured Intracranial Aneurysms Investigators, et al. Unruptured intracranial aneurysms: natural history, clinical outcome, and risks of surgical and endovascular treatment. Lancet. 2003;362(9378):103–10.

MIX
Papier aus verantwortungsvollen Quellen
Paper from responsible sources
FSC® C105338

If you have any concerns about our products,
you can contact us on
ProductSafety@springernature.com

In case Publisher is established outside the EU,
the EU authorized representative is:
Springer Nature Customer Service Center GmbH
Europaplatz 3, 69115 Heidelberg, Germany

Printed by Libri Plureos GmbH
in Hamburg, Germany